THE BRAINWASHING BOOK
Hypnotic, Erotic Behaviorism and Beyond

sleepingirl

Copyright © 2019 sleepingirl

All rights reserved. No part of this book may be reproduced or transmitted in any form or by any means, electronic or mechanical, including photocopying, recording, or by an information storage and retrieval system—except by a reviewer who may quote brief passages in a review or an educator who may quote brief passages and attribute content to the author—without permission in writing from the publisher.

ISBN-13: 978-1-7068-4689-5

Edited by Michal Daveed (GleefulAbandon), with help from sleepingirl and JusticeItself

Cover art and all formatting by sleepingirl

THE BRAINWASHING BOOK

For the hypnosis community: Maybe I really was born to meet you.

And for c.c.; my best friend, my brainwashed slave.

THE BRAINWASHING BOOK

CONTENTS

	Preface	viii
	Introduction: Erotic Behaviorism	xii
1	Introduction to Brainwashing	2
2	Methods for Brainwashing	12
3	Classical Conditioning	22
4	Operant Conditioning	34
5	Shaping	50
6	Hypnosis	56
7	Applications and Considerations	66
8	Tools	76
9	Fantasies and Scenes	102
10	Risky, Riskier, Riskiest	112
11	"Undoing" and "Deprogramming"	126
	In Conclusion	132
	Glossary	134
	Bibliography	138

THE BRAINWASHING BOOK

THE BRAINWASHING BOOK

PREFACE

I grew up with a true fetish for hypnosis and mind control—some of my earliest memories are of being confused and excited by these sorts of scenes in movies, TV, and books. In particular, I found myself drawn to the fantasy of having my control taken away from me, being lulled under the sway of another, giving up all of myself because I was hypnotized. As a child, I wondered if this was some unspoken desire that everyone shared, but I somehow knew innately that I wasn't supposed to talk about it. Growing older, I came to realize that I was alone, or not quite, as the internet eventually revealed to me—just in a small niche minority. I was so incredibly ashamed by what I felt were these bizarre tastes. I remember swearing to myself over and over that I'd keep it a secret forever.

But by 18, I found my curiosity for all of it grow insatiable, privately and obsessively doing research, listening to pre-recorded hypnosis files, watching video demonstrations, and eventually building up the courage to tell my girlfriend at the time about my proclivities. She was open to giving it a shot, with me as the hypnotist, and so for the first time, I stumbled my way through parroting how I thought a hypnotic induction was supposed to go. It was messy and it felt so embarrassing, but it was closer than I ever expected to get.

For a few years, I dabbled with hypnosis on both sides of the pocket watch in my vanilla relationships before finally taking my first steps towards meeting other hypnofetishists, initially online, and then going to real-life events, sharing space with like-minded people. It was an absolute dream come true, and it supercharged the way I learned about this fascinating thing that we all share. I heard stories like mine over and over and at last felt at home. I kept some of the shame as an exciting, transgressive feeling, but got braver about talking about it and especially doing it.

But no matter how much I played (and I played as though I was making up for lost time), I always wanted more, and found myself constantly yearning for those childhood fantasies of being completely taken, destroyed, reprogrammed—but now with a mirroring desire to do the same to someone of my own. And then, six years ago, I was entering into a D/s relationship and I remember telling my submissive partner what I wanted to eventually do. Her eyes went wide and she whispered privately to me, excited and nervous, "You can't say that! I mean, that's the hottest thing in the world, but you aren't allowed to say that kind of thing!"

My skills as a hypnotist grew exponentially as I had a partner who, while she wasn't a hypnofetishist, wanted the same things that I did. And they grew adjacently in a different way; I began to really focus on what "brainwashing" meant to us and how we could achieve it in a long-term, ethical, and committed relationship. We did it all in a sort of vacuum—at that time, people just weren't talking in depth about this kind of thing, and I always wished that there were more resources from which I could learn. Talking about our relationship always made people echo that, and so about two years ago, a little drunk after work and having a passionate conversation with my brainwashed slave, I said, "Fuck it," and opened a blank document and just started writing.

This book is one culmination of my ten years of practice thus far and my experience with "brainwashing" both as a hypnotist and subject. It contains no "101" hypnosis material—you won't find a description of how to do inductions or what hypnosis is. It is for the intermediate practitioner who is looking to learn not only about practical, consensual brainwashing, but useful psychological concepts and more advanced hypnotic discussion that informs everything that we all do. While it's written from the perspective of the hypnotist, I encourage subject-identified individuals to read it, as knowledge of the play that you desire to engage in is a key aspect of being able to consent to it and converse about it.

Brainwashing is a way of connecting intimately on levels that we sometimes have no proper frame of reference with which to handle. It is exciting, it is hot, and it is intellectually mesmerizing. If you learn just one thing, I will have succeeded in what I set out to do. I learned a lot just by writing it. I wrote this book for you—you who picked it up; you who had some interest in this crazy fantasy; you who were curious; you who had a journey just like I did, similar or different, that somehow brought you here.

Please enjoy it!

THE BRAINWASHING BOOK

INTRODUCTION: "EROTIC BEHAVIORISM"

Hypnosis itself can be better understood when there is context to why we do things the way that we do them, and I believe the same is true about conditioning and other areas of mind play. My own research into it has yielded a greater depth of knowledge on the "why," and consequently, on how to apply them erotically.

There are, of course, many, many brilliant scientists who have done so much research and discovery on the topics presented in this book. In psychology, so much blends together; to some degree as I talk about one thing, it is impossible to discuss without first considering how it is related to another, and so on. But as we are going to explore both classical conditioning and operant conditioning, it is prudent to reference two of the most influential people in these areas of research: Ivan Pavlov, and Burrhus Frederic Skinner, respectively.

These two men—and topics—are hugely important to a school of thought that was popular in the 20th century known as "behaviorism." Behaviorism is a sort of fusion of psychology and philosophy that has many different roots and variations. The general underlying principle that most behaviorists believed was that the behaviors of all organisms (including humans) are simply reflexes, learned from conditioning through interaction with their environment or a product of their personal history. Behaviorists were mainly concerned with the methodology of a "stimulus-response" system; that is, how behavior (or response) can be predicted when a stimulus is present. To some degree, behaviorists were interested in this type of "learning" above all else.

Pavlov, Skinner, and "Radical Behaviorism"

Ivan Pavlov (of the eponymous dogs) discovered that dogs' salivation in response to food was a reflexive behavior that fit neatly inside of the "stimulus-response" model, and that by presenting another stimulus (such as a bell), the dogs learned by association to have a conditioned response of salivating to it. Thus formed the basis for classical conditioning. This approach falls quite neatly into the stimulus-response theory, and his continued research into the concept of pairing stimuli through this type of conditioning was foundational for behaviorism.

On the other hand, B.F. Skinner is widely considered the father of operant conditioning; his research diverged from Pavlov in that he was interested in being able to control and shape behavior of organisms directly by applying reinforcements and punishments—"carrot and stick." Notably, while behaviorists before him were focused only on measurable, observable external events, in Skinner's philosophy of "radical behaviorism," he pioneered the idea that private events—internal thoughts and experiences— were also relevant to consider since they too were behaviors themselves (or things that affected them).

This was a game changer; in most behaviorist thought at the time, thoughts and feelings were seen as unscientific, and only external events were worthy or able to be studied. To some degree, this is true, and is in fact one of its biggest criticisms: How is it possible to accurately measure someone's thoughts and subjective experiences and therefore prove the effect it has on behavior? Even if they are reported by the subject verbally, this is just an interpretation or approximation; not empirical at all.

What we do in the erotic hypnosis community, however, relies heavily on these types of "unscientific" interactions. We are constantly attempting to synthesize our thoughts into speech so our partners may better understand what phenomena we are experiencing. Indeed, it's crucial to me to consider my partner's private internal experiences as something that influences them and their behavior, or to see them as malleable behaviors on their own. Whether or not I can study them objectively has little consequence to me; we come up with our own models of how to discuss this, and anecdotally it works as best it can for us.

The Human Caveat

Behaviorism sounds like a logical and attractive approach, and many of the experiments and findings (indeed, the theories of classical and operant conditioning themselves) are highly successful in predicting and shaping behavior. But while it is a helpful model and very interesting, and while I do believe that conditioning accounts for more than we often give it credit for, it is rather outdated. It is widely understood that there are many other factors to human development. In fact, one of the principles of some forms of behaviorism is that humans are not distinct from animals in the way that they learn or are conditioned. In his book, "Punished By Rewards" on the failings of so-called "pop behaviorism" in human society, Alfie Kohn was appalled by Skinner's idea of people as collections of behaviors. He notes with a tone of disbelief that Skinner wrote:

"I am sometimes asked, 'Do you think of yourself as you

think of the organisms you study?' The answer is yes. So far as I know, my behavior at any given moment has been nothing more than the product of my genetic endowment, my personal history, and the current setting . . . . If I am right about human behavior, I have written the autobiography of a nonperson."[1]

I am not as disgusted as Kohn seemed to be by this idea, but at the very least I can acknowledge that it might be troubling if taken too literally. There are different types of learning and an absurd amount of variables that influence humans and human behavior. This is no more apparent than when we are working as hypnotists; hypnosis works best when we are keenly aware that our partners' experiences depend on an innumerable amount of factors. Understanding them is a goal as important as achieving any of the erotic experiences we have planned.

Personally, I am very fond of the concept of behaviorism, even if I can easily accept that humans are absurdly complex. But what I really want to emphasize is that while thinking of your partner as a collection of responses and behaviors is a large swath of what we'll be exploring, I hope that we don't become so bogged down in that idea that we forget our partners are, in fact, human, and behaviorism does not tell a complete picture of the human mind. None of the techniques I'm introducing here and will be describing are quite as simplistic as they might seem—as easy as input-output, or stimulus-response, and I hope to make this clear in the text.

Erotic Behaviorism

I'm quite taken by the behaviorist approach and its

---

[1] Kohn, A. (2018). *Punished by Rewards: The Trouble with Gold Stars, Incentive Plans, A's, Praise, and Other Bribes.* Houghton Mifflin Harcourt Trade & Reference Publishers.

impact on psychology. In fact, Skinner's "nonperson" comment even fuels some of the erotic appeal of it. The foundation for this book is derived in large part from this school of thought, with my own caveats and alterations through experience and belief. "Behaviorism," in the way that I see it, puts an emphasis on how organisms learn and grow, and the ability to have a certain mindset in how we view ourselves and others as (at least partially) products of stimuli and our responses to them.

    This is very much in my wheelhouse and how I view human interaction as a whole: "Conditioning is learning," "Conditioning is a mindset," "Conditioning is everywhere," all concepts that we will be exploring. This is how I effectively brainwash: By learning how to understand responses and control them to fit my goals, as well as being open to exploring the unknown and unpredictable. I do this with the understanding that my partners are complex and influenced by their own motivations, histories, thoughts, experiences, and more. I do this by learning about them as people, and using all of my knowledge about them to shape them. I use hypnosis as a way to communicate and enhance our intimate experiences; intimacy on some level (whether intellectual, casual, playful, physical, or otherwise) is a "must."

This is my form of behaviorism: Erotic behaviorism. The ability to confidently yet cautiously view my partner as a hugely complex and flawed stimulus-response system, the ability to be able to pay attention and connect as a tool to better shape them for my desires, the ability to acknowledge all of our shared history, the ability to learn about their internal and subjective experiences as a way to "improve" their behavior. When this philosophy is merged with hypnosis, it feels like anything is possible.

THE BRAINWASHING BOOK

CHAPTER 1: INTRODUCTION TO BRAINWASHING

"Brainwashing" is a word that is as alluring as it is frightening, full of mystery and hidden knowledge. For some, it has negative, perhaps political associations; for others, a deep, intense eroticism. Often, it is more complicated than just one or the other, and perhaps it also evokes a certain curiosity, of wanting to dig into "what," "how," and "why." For the purpose of this book, we'll be talking about brainwashing as a positive thing with a particularly broad kinky definition: A sexy form of play that allows us to set and achieve goals using a variety of well-known psychological methods and deeply enjoy the process and fantasies behind it.

Even within that more narrowed scope, there are a lot of ideas that the word "brainwashing" might bring to mind. Some people imagine technologically complex machines doing some unknowable work, or perhaps a powerfully manipulative person taking and shaping a victim. For some of us, brainwashing has always been at the core of our sexuality—the idea of inciting change or being changed, temporarily or permanently, involving some loss of self or slow, insidious takeover. Perhaps the word "control" plays a big part in all of it. Within the framework of hypnosis or mind control fantasies, brainwashing often lies tantalizingly at the crux of the two, and beyond.

What Is Brainwashing?

Words, tricky as they are, have different definitions for everyone; the concept of "connotation" is notoriously important for what we do with kink and hypnosis. It defines how well we succeed in giving ourselves and our partners what we want; the desire to do "erotic hypnosis" can have so many different meanings to different people that it's imperative to discuss further and dig into what that entails practically. Some of the most enlightening and enriching conversations come from sitting down with others and comparing our histories and experiences, which often involves discussing personal connotations in one way or another for the things that we do.

That's perfectly fine: This book will explore a goal-oriented approach to brainwashing, and before even taking your first steps into the "hows," you must first begin to get an understanding of what that word means to you.

Getting Started: General Versus Specific

Sometimes even in self-reflection, it is difficult to nail down exactly what such a generalized term really means. Many find it challenging to answer questions such as, "What does it mean to be brainwashed?" Or, "What makes a brainwashed slave/partner/label-of-choice?" These are not only very broad, generalized questions, but they focus on goals that are more long-term; ideas about perfection, and constant, daily growth to something larger.

It's helpful in mental exercises such as this one to focus on specifics; "I want my partner to…" Fold the laundry every day? Desire to please you? Feel controlled? Maybe something even more specific, like rolling their eyes up when they go into trance. These ideas may come naturally, or may come from "research" (perhaps looking at porn or reading erotica), or be shamelessly borrowed in flattering imitation. It's OK to glean inspiration wherever you find it. Think of these specific "short-term" goals as leading to the long-term ones.

Consider the sentence, "Someone who is brainwashed..." and begin to fill in the blanks. It's OK if some of the ideas that you come up with don't apply to everyone or every situation. This type of brainstorming is all about being a starting point for exploring possibilities. You don't have to know exactly what the perfect brainwashed slave is from day one. It's a fun exercise where you can fantasize freely; it's helpful for some people to write things down and organize them, but the idea of this is to get your brain moving in a productive direction. Oftentimes, these ideas will come along the way and as part of this process of growing together with your partner. Goals like these are not immutable; flexibility and understanding that both you and your partner are humans, constantly changing, is a big part of what we'll be exploring.

Once you have some concept of some of the "whats" that you are looking for, it is helpful as well to dig into the "whys." In some ways, this is about exploring your motivation and may require a little soul-searching: Perhaps this is something about which you have always fantasized, but why? What about it makes it so attractive? Is there a feeling of power associated with being able to do this? Do you like the idea of helplessness? Or perhaps it is the idea of a long session of mind-melting change. This idea of being able to begin to understand "why" you do what you do can help to guide and ensure that when you start to play with achieving your goals, you are not so focused on the process of achieving the "what" that you lose sight of what really makes it good for you and your partner.

Negotiation

This is not a process that you have to—or should—approach alone. Some of the most powerful brainstorming is with our intimate partners; they are other human minds to bounce off of and explore, and their input is valuable, especially when we are talking about a common interest.

Talking with your partner about what brainwashing means to you as well as them is significant on several fundamental levels, the first of which is an ethical one. There are many models in hypnosis and general kink for "negotiating": Ensuring that all parties involved are consenting to and understand the depth of what is involved. The idea of brainwashing someone is no exception to the category of things that should be negotiated in this way—a full and clear understanding of what everyone is thinking as far as possibilities is enormously important.

As we'll be exploring, the risks of these activities and what they encompass in general are extremely broad, so in many cases, it's impossible to come into a discussion with a checklist and have that be complete. The best we can do is be as open as we can, especially in the beginning, and certainly throughout the relationship about where everyone is at in terms of comfort and knowledge. Where are the boundaries? What aspects of life will be potentially affected? Even if everyone is doing their best to keep the brainwashing contained, is it acceptable that there is a chance that there will be bleedover? What behavioral changes are safe and acceptable, and are there any that are 100% off limits? Is it ok that you're not able to fully negotiate everything in advance?

Some people may pick up this book in the hope of grasping immediately what is acceptable, how far brainwashing can go, how much it reaches into our lives, and exactly how to negotiate about it. There is no easy answer for this. However, learning what is presented here will give you a better grasp on how to talk about these topics in a more informed and mature way and hopefully lead into a deeper comprehension of how to effectively negotiate these techniques to the best of your ability and to a level that is mutually acceptable. Being able to properly negotiate something absolutely requires understanding it first.

We should ideally respect and want what's best for our partners, and it is imperative that they have a say—and an enthusiastic "yes!"—in the fun we intend to have together. Brainwashing can be a heavy-duty activity, with potential for risks and real life changes, and it can't be stressed enough that these discussions are morally very important. It may also be helpful to have safewords (agreed-upon words with predetermined meaning, like "all play must stop" or "pause and check in") to ensure that both parties have a mechanism to halt a scene or have a power-neutral discussion.

Of course, in some relationship models, it is pre-negotiated that play on this level is allowable with a certain amount of secrecy. This can certainly be a fun idea—changing someone without their knowledge. Some relationships eschew the idea of a detailed negotiation in favor of feeling everything out as they go. There may be quite a bit of wiggle room for this. This too is acceptable; everyone negotiating to the level that is mutually comfortable for them and their partners is the ideal.

Keep Talking With Your Partner

There are several reasons that it's beneficial to have these conversations from time to time, regardless of relationship style. The tool of simply setting an intention can be very powerful and motivating. In dog training, we have to rely on nonverbal methods for training, because dogs don't understand what we're saying. With humans, we don't have this problem. And in many hypnotic relationships, where there is a desire to please the hypnotist, dominant, or "brainwasher," understanding the intent of their partner is something that begins to create change all on its own. As we'll be exploring later, there are many factors that influence the nebulous concept of "conditionability"—not a technical term, but a concept worthy of exploration—and for many, the associations involved with understanding what you really want can be very strong.

There is another concept besides ethics and efficacy that should be mentioned here—the idea of progressing a relationship through exploring. Some of our fondest memories with our partners might be excited, engaged, perhaps late-night conversations about our mutual desires and interests. This is one of the ways we grow together and learn about each other, and that feeling of deep, personal understanding (and of being understood) is a common human need. (No better discussed here than in countless songs, poems, and media; for a fun, musical example, look no further than the classic "Getting to Know You" from "The King and I.")

These conversations don't have to be explicit and fabricated "we need to sit down and talk" moments. Some of the best mutual learning happens spontaneously and organically, throughout the course of a relationship, no matter the form, whether you live together with your partner or they are across the world. Big revelations sometimes happen in the most unlikely of times and places; having good communication skills and habits with your partner is tantamount to doing the really good, intimate stuff.

Potential Goals

What are some ideas to get started on what it means to be brainwashed? Here are a few examples.

- Enjoyment of selfless sexual acts
    - "I want my partner to want to do things for me sexually and get off on it to the point that it is its own reward."

- Acting in ways that are personally sexually provocative
    - "I want my partner to be as attractive to me as possible." Whether there's a certain phrase they say that always gets you going, or you like the way their eyes flutter sometimes in trance, you can encourage these behaviors and the general mindset of wanting to turn you on.
- Inclination to share vanilla hobbies and interests
    - "Whether it's about where we go out to dinner, what TV series we watch, or what game we play online together, I desire agreeableness and genuine delight in my choices."
- Responsiveness to—and enjoyment of—conditioning
    - "I like behavior modification for its own sake, and I want my partner to like it too—and be really good at it."
- Responsiveness to—and enjoyment of—hypnosis
    - "I want my partner to be quickly and easily responsive to my suggestions and trance."
- Drive for anticipatory service
    - "I value service: Acts that do something for me in some way that make my life easier." Sometimes it is nice to directly order service ("Go get me a glass of water"), but it's balanced with being able to rely on tasks getting done or someone anticipating your needs.
- Faith in being brainwashed
    - "I want my partner to proudly proclaim, 'Yes, I am brainwashed!' and truly believe it." This is both very erotic in its own right as well as is a powerful mindset which helps to facilitate further change.

- A sense of feeling "owned" or controlled
  - "I want my partner to feel like I possess them fully, I help shape them, I help to define who they are, and that they belong to me." D/s ownership dynamics fit neatly into brainwashing.
- Inclination towards being playful or "bratty"
  - "I want my partner to know just how to provoke me in a positive way to get my attention." For those that enjoy that sort of spiritedness and fun punishment!
- Compelled obedience
  - "I want my partner to be driven to obey me." It is one thing to want to listen and obey—perhaps it's another to feel it in their bones.
- Change in perception
  - "I want my partner to always see me as super sexy and smart."

These are just a few general ideas to get us going. Over the course of brainwashing in a relationship, we often develop preferences and tastes based on how we grow together that we can work on applying if we so desire.

Notice that some of these examples have outward actions associated with them (like sexual servitude), and some are more about internal changes (personal belief in brainwashedness). If you start to give thought to it, it's not that each item falls into one category or the other, but more so that there are levels of internal and external aspects to each of them. For example, in anticipatory service, the external actions are constant, but are being driven by a powerful internal motivation: To want to please and learn more about how to do it more effectively in this way.

Considering the hidden, private events and behaviors inside your partner is just as important as affecting outward change. To some degree, the internal influences the external, and the external influences the internal. The act of repeating a mantra can potentially affect your partner's thinking (as we'll explore), and if that mantra causes them to have internal desires to sexually serve you, those private thoughts may cause them to act differently around you, perhaps more seductively, submissively, or otherwise.

The Unspoken Goal

The biggest, overarching goal in a relationship is to have fun. Different parts and pieces of all of this will be differently attractive to everyone, and a key takeaway from it should be that you both "learn how to learn" what works best for you in terms of efficacy and hotness. This might mean staying really rigid to your goal-setting at times while exploring nebulously at others. Perhaps instead of rushing through progress, you slow down and savor it, because it's the process itself of being changed by another person that is one of the sexiest aspects of it all.

There are all sorts of different ways to apply what is in the book, and this is only one perspective on how to use several well-established and layman-explained psychological concepts. Keep an open mind and remember that in the end, this is all about having a good time and creating mutually enjoyable experiences.

THE BRAINWASHING BOOK

CHAPTER 2: METHODS FOR BRAINWASHING

So naturally, the next big question is, "How do we achieve some or all of these goals?" Of course, hypnosis is a fun tool to use and one of the focal points of this book. But it's not strictly the whole of what we do, even if we're not aware of it. This book is going to introduce a few key concepts that don't necessarily rely on hypnosis. At the same time as exploring them as tools for brainwashing as a whole, keep in mind that effective hypnosis, in many cases, necessarily relies on them.

Conditioning and Hypnosis

The bread and butter of what we'll be talking about in terms of brainwashing, effective hypnosis, and behavior modification is conditioning. Specifically, operant and classical conditioning, which are distinct in both history and functionality, but related practically in terms of shaping all organisms (including people).

- "Classical" or "Pavlovian" conditioning uses

association and pairing stimuli to change behavior—like bells with drooling dogs.
- "Operant" or "instrumental" conditioning is what comes to mind when we think of traditional "training," like dog training or child rearing; using reinforcement and punishment to encourage or discourage behaviors.

Both of these are big topics on their own but fall under a larger umbrella: Conditioning is a form of learning. Learning can be defined as "A relatively lasting change in behavior that is the result of experience"[2]—and maybe this sounds exactly like what we are looking to grasp. The types of conditioning we'll be working with are part of something slightly more specific, called "associative learning." Associative learning also has an interesting definition: "Any learning process in which a new response becomes associated with a particular stimulus."[3] So, by using context, associative learning is any somewhat lasting change in behavior resulting from a response being associated with a stimulus.

Conditioning is not only a tool to intentionally change your partner to be more desirable, it is one of the primary ways that humans and other organisms grow and learn in their lives. We learn certain behaviors are acceptable through environmental factors; you touch the stove as a child and quickly learn that something that hot is not for touching—maybe even develop a fear about it. The positive or negative reactions of our peers in high school sometimes dictated what we considered to be the right way to dress or act. When you have a great, intimate experience with a partner, it influences your thoughts and behavior; you may

---

[2] Cherry, K. (2019, September 24). The Psychology of How People Learn. Retrieved from http://www.verywellmind.com/what-is-learning-2795332.
[3] Britannica, T. E. of E. (n.d.). Associative learning. Retrieved from http://www.britannica.com/topic/associative-learning.

want to do more and you've built an association with them as a person who makes you feel good.

Conditioning as a Mindset

One of the most important concepts in this book is that conditioning—associative learning—is something we are doing and experiencing absolutely all the time. When you respond to your partner with genuine enthusiasm, you are shaping their behavior. When you finally call your nagging relatives and they pick up and testily ask why you don't call more often, you are being shaped in a very different direction. Associations are paired absolutely everywhere as a function of how we learn.

From this perspective, brainwashing is a mindset not only for the brainwashed partner, but for the partner doing the brainwashing. Having the understanding that so much of what we do is influenced by our responses to each other is immensely powerful. There is a mindfulness involved in the kind of attentiveness we're talking about. That kind of deep awareness on our own behavior around other people, especially the partners we care about, is key to effectively controlling and changing them in desirable ways. It is something that becomes natural over time; becoming more mindful of how we treat others and mindful of how others might perceive our actions and reactions. Understanding that this is one of the primary ways that your partner learns and being able to guide that process is very powerful.

Perhaps this view of conditioning seems like an unfamiliar commitment; in some ways, it is, but it is not so different from how we think and interact normally. When we talk to others, we generally try to have some understanding of how our speech and actions will be taken. We know that some topics or advice may be received better than others. We know that if we choose to blow someone off, it may be taken negatively. The first part of this mindset is just this, something akin to a very basic empathy: Being able to understand how our behavior is seen by others. The second part may take a bit of thinking and practice—the shift towards considering what behaviors we may be encouraging, discouraging, or associating—but this quickly becomes natural.

Having this particular knowledge that conditioning is everywhere will improve your interpersonal relationships in general, as well as allow you a far more broad and tangible sense of control when using it intentionally to shape a partner for erotic purposes. Sharing an awareness with your partner that your intent is to change them over time—and that you are actively doing so—is very hot. It takes mundane moments like saying "thank you" and elevates them to a level of sexy play. This is a way to incorporate more of the eroticism in your daily lives.

Hypnosis

This book assumes some basic knowledge of hypnosis, and will be referencing hypnotic techniques in conjunction with conditioning. Hypnosis isn't necessary by any means for some of the goal-oriented conditioning we're exploring here, but it is truly a useful tool on its own and can be very effective as an addition to it. Hypnotic techniques can, for example, speed up the processes of conditioning when applied correctly and attentively, and make various aspects much easier.

Besides being useful, hypnosis is a very sexy activity in and of itself to a lot of people. For many, "brainwashing" necessarily includes hypnosis as part of the trope. Hypnosis also allows us to do imaginative "scenes"—erotic sessions of play—that transcend reality and create absolutely magical experiences. When used properly, it's a tool not only for change, but for intimacy and connection.

Many phenomena and processes in hypnosis "work" because of operant and classical conditioning. We are constantly trying to encourage desired hypnotic behavior from our partners by using praise and pleasure—"That's right," "It feels good to sink, doesn't it?" Classical conditioning and pairing stimuli (e.g., a snap of the fingers with the feeling of dropping deep into trance) is at the core of creating effective triggers and responses. Even the word "deeper" holds as much weight as it does because of how we (and our partners) have been conditioned to understand it. We wouldn't be able to do hypnosis in the way that we do it now if humans didn't grow and process through associative learning. And of course there is the flipside of this: It describes why we don't want to do certain things with hypnosis, such as inadvertently discouraging responsiveness, or creating negative associations with our play. Part of this book will be about exploring how to apply these tools to make our hypnosis better: By understanding them as parts of hypnosis itself.

What Are the Risks?

As with most any activities we engage in over the course of our lives, there are risks involved in approaching this kind of play. In the kink community, there are several acronyms that serve as a model for this—one of them is "RACK," or, "Risk-Aware Consensual Kink." Breaking this down, it tells us that there are risks in everything we do, and the key to more informed play—hopefully safer play—is to recognize the risks, try to mitigate them when we can, and ensure that our partners are on the same page and are able to give their informed consent.

With brainwashing in particular, the risks are heavily dependent on our personal goals. Try to explore and think carefully and critically about what potential risks your goals might have on you and your partner. And of course, risks do not only apply to the bottom; they are not a one-way street. We will discuss specific risk-assessment and mitigation in further depth in Chapter 10, but here are a few possibilities:

- Dependency or "neediness/clinginess"
    - This seems to be one of the biggest aspects of riskiness in this type of play; we are all familiar with clingy and dependent behavior, where someone constantly wants or needs attention, time, and energy. The kind of attentiveness required in brainwashing in the way we describe it tends to exacerbate this and create it where there previously may have been none.
- Falling in love
    - Over time, the intensity of this type of play can create a very intimate bond. "Friends with benefits" relationships are famously hard to maintain; lots of people find it challenging to stick with something platonic when sex is involved, not to mention brainwashing. Nobody is immune to strong emotions.
- Inability to trust objective decision-making
    - For an example, you may not be able to ask your partner, "Does this look good on me?" and expect an empirical response; sometimes you may even get the very flattering but unhelpful, "You always look good," complete with an adoring look and a wistful sigh. This is great, and if a piece of clothing really does look hideous, your partner may not be blind to it, but nevertheless this is potentially a concern, especially if you are asking about something more important than the way you dress. This becomes especially problematic when you consider that you may not be able to negotiate with them in an uninfluenced state.

- Complications with the relationship ending
    - It is a good idea to have some sort of contingency plan for if a relationship goes south or ends abruptly, but it is not always possible to be prepared for every circumstance, and often, that preparation is not as simple as we'd like it to be. We can't wave a magic wand and erase all the history that we have with each other.
- Constant desire for escalation
    - What do you do when you or your partner always seem to want more—and more intensity? It's not always possible to escalate the feeling of "potency" of what we're doing, and it may not always be healthy, either. Making choices about how and when to handle this can be tricky.

If some or all of these sound familiar, or you think to yourself, "But these can happen in any relationship!" then you are quickly picking up on this concept we keep coming back to: There is conditioning in almost everything we do. Conditioning is not a new idea or something unique to brainwashing. The difference is using it intentionally to achieve goals. In some ways, these risks are heightened from a non-brainwashing relationship in that we are, to some degree, utilizing conditioning more effectively. From another perspective, the awareness of these risks and the ability to see conditioning as it happens makes some of them easier to mitigate—but not necessarily eliminate—when we are able to do so.

This book is not intended to give solid answers on how to fix these issues; that would be impossible. The best way to address any risks within a relationship is to have open and detailed discussions of how best to handle them with the specific people involved. Every relationship is different. It's also valuable to understand that sometimes, we can't mitigate risks as fully as we might like—we just have to accept them as a part of what we're doing. Accepting them means that we have to account for the possibility that they happen. Understanding more about how conditioning works in an intimate, purposeful partnership allows us to make personalized choices on how to proceed and how to handle that.

Time and Energy Commitment: "24/7"

Brainwashing, in the model we are using, is a commitment in the same way that being in a relationship is a commitment. If conditioning is something that is happening to us constantly, then acknowledging and paying attention to that is part of that commitment. For some people, this fits into the category of a "24/7" relationship: We are affecting our partners with what we do in ways that may influence their lives at any time.

As will be discussed as we go on, being lax in the wrong ways on conditioning can inhibit change and growth and cause confusion. "Constant vigilance" is a good phrase; it is our job to be attentive and responsive to our partners, reinforce when needed, recondition responses when needed, and most centrally, be ready to have conversations about our partners' feelings or potential concerns.

In the BDSM and kink world, "24/7" is a marker generally used to differentiate relationships where couples are only kinky "in the bedroom" from those who have aspects of dominance and submission (D/s) every day. Whether or not someone terms their relationship as 24/7 is highly about personal view and preference. This is not to suggest that all brainwashing relationships are inherently a 24/7 D/s dynamic, but some prefer to define their own relationships as such because it allows them to acknowledge the work they are putting in at all times and the change, growth, and learning that is happening every day.

Of course, we have to acknowledge that we are human

and there are times when we will not be "on." We are not perfect, and neither are our partners. Sometimes we don't have the energy to pay as close attention or condition behavior. This is normal, but good to be aware of in and of itself; we should try to ensure that we all have reasonable expectations of our habits and levels of activity. Sometimes we are actively messaging our partners, or making dates every week, and sometimes we're just not up for it. Our partners, too, are not going to be available to us or in a perfect mood at all times. This is normal relationship stuff, being able to manage excitement, disappointment, and other expectations without them becoming world-ending. It is not that we are no longer 24/7 if we miss an opportunity or let something slide. We are 24/7 because we acknowledge our humanness and communicate about it.

Think About These Guidelines

How do we know if something is problematic? Of course, there isn't a black-and-white answer, as everyone's lines for what is acceptable are going to be different and may change over time. However, there are some general guidelines and cautions to consider:

- Encourage them to keep in touch with their friends and family
    - Relationships become incredibly problematic when one partner neglects their life responsibilities, and especially if that includes communication with their loved ones. There shouldn't be any circumstances where they are discouraged from interacting with people who are positive influences in their lives.
- Make sure they can always express what they are feeling
    - We need our partners' genuine expression

just as much as they do. It allows us to make decisions, whether that's mutual or consensually one-sided, to the best of our abilities. We must be able to trust that they will talk to us if they really enjoy something or if something is a problem for them, or just generally being able to speak their minds.

- Advocate for agency and self-sufficiency whenever possible
    - One of the best ways to mitigate the risk of dependency is ensuring that we cultivate a sense of agency and independence in our partners. This might include concepts like making sure they're capable of making decisions on their own, or that they have strong self image.
- Respond to discomfort
    - If our partners come to us with something that is bothering them, it's our job to respond to it. Likewise, if we notice something that they're not saying, it's our job to ask and do what we can to alleviate problems. We want enjoyable and harmonious relationships, and especially when there is a power imbalance like in D/s or brainwashing, a lot of responsibility falls on us.

CHAPTER 3: CLASSICAL CONDITIONING

Ivan Pavlov did not set out to discover the concept of classical conditioning when he was working with dogs. He was, in fact, studying digestion. But he noticed that the dogs would salivate when food was present, but saw something curious: The dogs would salivate when they saw an assistant in a white lab coat enter the room, even if they weren't bringing any food.

This, he theorized, was because the dogs had learned an association between the assistants' presence and the food, and therefore the response had been conditioned into them. His began doing research to try to discern more about the nature of how these responses were acquired. In a well-known example, he played the sounds of various noise-making objects—most famously a bell—before presenting the dogs with food. After a few repetitions, the dogs would salivate when the bell was played, despite food not being present. This is the essence of classical conditioning—pairing a stimulus that evokes a response to a neutral one, such that the neutral stimulus evokes the same (or a similar) response to the original stimulus.

Definitions

There are several elements at play here when broken down.

- Unconditioned stimulus (food): A stimulus that evokes a response
- Unconditioned response (salivating to the food): The natural response to the unconditioned stimulus
- Conditioned stimulus (bell): A stimulus that is generally neutral
- Conditioned response (salivating to the bell): The learned response to the conditioned stimulus

The basic idea of classical conditioning is that things can be associated through a well-known process; certainly this has many applications erotically. Getting orgasms on command is the holy grail for some people, and many do it even without hypnosis. Classical conditioning is the name for the principle that makes that happen; a careful, planned association between, for example, a countdown (conditioned stimulus) and someone masturbating (unconditioned stimulus), or the tone of a bell (conditioned stimulus) with reaching that edge (conditioned response).

Certainly, then, when we add hypnosis into the mix, we get something immensely versatile and powerful. In the orgasm example, we could take advantage of the power of the mind and have the subject vividly imagine self-stimulation—then there may be less of a hurdle to get to hands-free orgasms. We also have the ability to directly suggest associations. When we think about achieving hypnotic orgasms, classical conditioning comes into play more than we might expect. Subjects who have a strong association with, for example, that countdown and deep pleasure, will generally have better and faster learning responses.

Of course, this is the big, flashy kind of classical conditioning. The reality is that our lives are full of these conditioned responses. When you get a message or a phone call and your heart starts to pound even before you know who it's from; when you walk into the doctor's office and feel nervous, or when you drive to a friend's house and feel excited.

And just as much as your cat is conditioned to expect food at a certain time because of your routine, you are conditioned to feel like you need to feed them. Conditioning doesn't only go in one direction—it isn't so much that one person is conditioning another, but that associations are being built (and as we'll learn later with operant conditioning, reinforcements given) in many ways at once that affect all parties involved.

Classical conditioning is something that you can do outside of the context of hypnosis, but that doesn't mean that you have to sit down and ring a bell every time that your partner is masturbating. It may be more helpful to be focused on the ways that you can use your knowledge of this principle to enhance your hypnosis, how you talk to them, and how you act around them. We can think very much about what associations our partners have with certain activities, spaces, and words. As we'll be exploring, classical conditioning is some of the foundation for why certain parts of hypnosis work in the way that they work.

Extinction in Classical Conditioning

Before we dig into methods, there is a part of classical conditioning (and operant conditioning, as we'll see later) that is critical for controlling and understanding responses. This is known as "extinction," and it refers to the concept that after a period of time of presenting the conditioned stimulus without the unconditioned stimulus being present, the conditioned stimulus will eventually stop eliciting the conditioned response. So, even though the bell will make the dogs drool, if the bell is rung enough times without the food being periodically introduced, the sound will at some point no longer cause them to salivate. The response is then considered to be extinguished (or extinct).

There is no set interval for how quickly a response will become extinct; it is dependent on far too many factors to be able to predict. The most reliable thing to do is to carefully monitor our partners' progress and responses. There has also been research done on persistence of response that corresponds to how the response was conditioned in the first place, which we will explore in the next section. This also gives us a clear indication of what to consider in terms of what this means for us practically: We may need to periodically re-pair stimuli and responses in order for them to have longevity. This applies to hypnosis, as well.

Not only is this important for those of us looking to change and control behavior, but it is important for our partners' well-being. Extinction can be a stressful process; suddenly losing the desired response over time can feel like failure. In hypnosis, we can see this in trigger responses: There is a notable feeling of disappointment for many subjects if a trigger has faded from disuse. It feels like something isn't working. In animals, we have a limit on what we can do if we want a learned response to go away. But in humans, it's necessary to remember that we can verbally understand each other. Stating the desire to abandon a response is something that will get you a long way and help to avoid the feeling of letting someone down, which is a hard burden for anyone to bear. In many cases, a gentle statement of intent in this way will do a lot of the work for you for extinguishing a learned behavior; at the very least, it motivates your partner to change in the direction that you desire.

Of course, even the fact that a response has begun to disappear is natural, since extinction is a known phenomenon. Sharing this knowledge with your partner is extremely helpful as well for someone who is experiencing extinction; they are not failing, they are going through a natural process.

Spontaneous Recovery / "Reconditioning"

Additionally, just because a behavior is thought to be extinguished doesn't mean it won't reemerge. For example, perhaps Pavlov's dogs were presented with the bell for a long enough period of time that they stopped drooling when they heard it. If he gave a period of rest after the response had become extinct, and then rang the bell again, the dogs may very well have started salivating again.

Extinction is tricky and unpredictable, not only because it is generally an unwanted outcome, but because it is impossible to rely on as a sign that conditioning is "gone." It is not as simple as the idea that conditioned behaviors have vanished, but it is not as simple as them persisting, either. The reality tends to be somewhere in the middle: Conditioned responses will absolutely fade naturally over time if they aren't being kept up somehow, but it's possible they may be kicked up in the future.

Some of this has to do with whether or not the response is suggested or "renewed" in some way; in humans this can be as simple as being reminded of the response. A subject who was conditioned to feel pleasure at the snap of your fingers might feel that response wane to nothing over time. There's potential for them to be caught off guard by a loud snap that re-triggers that response… or you could help it along by preceding your snap with something like, "Remember what it used to feel like when I snapped my fingers?" That's phrased as a suggestion, of course, but anything that brings to mind the original response might help to recondition it.

"Reconditioning" is sort of a misnomer, as it doesn't function any differently than conditioning in the first place. But if you do decide to try to pick a response back up after it's been gone or extinct, there are a couple things to consider. There is no right or wrong answer that applies to every situation of how to best go about doing this. You might think about following similar steps to what you did beforehand, which could have pros and cons: Maybe the steps are familiar in a positive way, or they remind your partner unpleasantly of when they lost the response. Conversely, if you train a response in a totally new way, it might be very effective, or more of a challenge to do something completely different. Oftentimes the answer lies somewhere in the middle of these two approaches. Making decisions with the information that you have available to you as well as being flexible is the best option.

Timing and Methods of Pairing

Practically, there are several different ways to associate and condition responses using classical conditioning. Each has a different method of implementation and variations on responsiveness. Much of this has to do with how we time the introduction of each stimulus.

Forward Conditioning

In forward conditioning, the conditioned stimulus is presented before the unconditioned stimulus. The bell is rung, then the dog is given food, resulting in the dog salivating at the bell. Forward conditioning is the most effective method; that is, it generally takes less time to do an initial pairing and generally the responses are more persistent. There is also further variance of timing in forward conditioning.

- In "delay" conditioning, the presentation of the conditioned stimulus overlaps with the unconditioned stimulus. The bell is rung first, but while the tone is still sounding the dog is given

food.
- In "trace" conditioning, the presentation of the conditioned stimulus does not overlap with the unconditioned stimulus. The bell is rung first, and after the tone has sounded, the dog is given food.

Simultaneous conditioning

In simultaneous conditioning, the conditioned stimulus is presented at the same time as the unconditioned stimulus. The bell is rung at the same time that the dog is given food, resulting in the dog salivating at the bell. While this is a very common thought process of how to condition a behavior, it is not the most effective, and we'll explore why (in many trials, it fails to produce a result at all.[4])

Second-Order Conditioning

In second-order conditioning, a primary conditioned stimulus is paired with an unconditioned stimulus, resulting in a conditioned response. Then, a secondary conditioned stimulus is paired with the first one, resulting in the secondary stimulus eliciting the conditioned response. The bell is rung just before the dog is given food, resulting in the dog salivating at the bell. Then, the sound of a metronome is played just before the sound of the bell, resulting in the metronome ultimately making the dog salivate.

Temporal Conditioning

In temporal conditioning, the unconditioned stimulus is presented at regular intervals, resulting in a conditioned response at regular intervals. The dog is given food at a certain time each day, resulting in salivation (or begging for

---

[4] Forms of Pavlovian Conditioning. (n.d.). Retrieved from http://www.indiana.edu/~p1013447/dictionary/pavfrm.htm.

food) at that time of day.

Backwards Conditioning

In backwards conditioning, the unconditioned stimulus follows the conditioned stimulus. The dog is given food, and then the bell is rung. Backwards conditioning is rarely effective, but has to do with the conditioned stimulus "predicting" the end of the unconditioned stimulus.

Factors That Affect Classical Conditioning

Of course, none of this happens in a vacuum. This makes sense; humans are hugely complex beings with dynamic lives and motivations. There are many variables that impact how classical conditioning works, as well as the effectiveness of pairing and how persistent some of these responses might be.

Stimulus Generalization

Stimulus generalization refers to the tendency for exposure to things similar to the conditioned stimulus to produce similar responses. For example, if your partner is conditioned to bark at the sound of a certain dog clicker, they may feel the urge to bark at the sound of a finger snap, or at the sound of a different clicker. It's for this reason that even if we try to be very, very specific with our conditioned responses (or triggers), recognition of the stimulus may be too fast for them to discern the difference.

Stimulus Discrimination

Stimulus discrimination, on the other hand, is the ability to distinguish between a stimulus that elicits a response and one that doesn't. This can be learned; in the previous example with the clicker, you can repeat the sound and reward responsiveness to it while not rewarding responses to other, similar sounds. Over time, and with persistence, your partner will tend to respond less to the similar sounds and more only to the original clicker.

Latent Inhibition

Latent inhibition is the concept that a stimulus that is familiar to the subject tends to take longer to associate meaning to than one that is not. So, if you are trying to condition your partner to feel pleasure whenever their childhood alarm clock goes off in the morning, it may take more persistence than if you bought them a new one with a new sound. Theoretically, this makes sense; the old alarm clock already has other longstanding associations with it.

Prediction Theory (Expectation)

While the foundation for classical conditioning is association, the pairing between stimuli isn't the whole of why we get the responses we get. In some models and discussions, one of the other key concepts relies on the idea that the presence of the conditioned stimulus "predicts" the arrival of the unconditioned stimulus. That is, the dog's brain has learned to expect food when the bell is rung, and that's from where the conditioned response comes.

This is a little bit of a subtle distinction, but there are several conclusions we can draw from this. For example, when we talk about how to pair responses in the first place, it becomes clear why forward conditioning (preceding the response) is one of the more effective and persistent methods; forward conditioning is all about prediction and expectation. While it seems logical in some ways that simultaneous conditioning (pairing at the same time) would be the quickest way to pair responses, it's been proven time and time again in trials that forward conditioning have the fastest and the most lasting associations, likely because of this concept of prediction.

Prediction theory also serves to explain extinction—if the bell isn't followed by food frequently enough, the brain learns that food isn't coming and stops making the response. When we think about persistence in responses, this is relevant to consider—what is the necessary amount of pairing that's needed to keep our subject expecting the response? As we've discussed, extinction can be avoidable with the right amount of upkeep and maintenance.

Belongingness

Some things pair better with others. The prevalent non-sexy example of this is in what's called "taste-aversion"—you get sick after eating a burger, and you immediately develop a distaste for burgers… and a persistent one, at that. It turns out that tastes are easily associated with illness. For a more fun example, many of us are familiar with the feeling of getting turned on when we see a certain sex toy, or pocket watch, or spiral that has relevance and history to us.

The reality is that some conditioned stimuli pair more effectively with certain unconditioned stimuli but not others, and vice versa, depending on whether or not there is a preexisting relationship between these two things. From a paper on conditioning in advertising, "Kim et al. (1998) found that if a CS and US have little or no pre-experimental conceptually based relationship with each other, classical conditioning can still occur as long as the subject does not hold any beliefs about the stimulus that might preclude conditioning."[5]

For this reason, it's wise to consider what associations you or your partner might have with a specific stimulus already. What does it symbolize? What memories and feelings does it already evoke? Is there already a response

---

[5] Schachtman, T. R., Walker, J., & Fowler, S. (2011). Effects of Conditioning in Advertising. *Associative Learning and Conditioning Theory*. doi: 10.1093/acprof:oso/9780199735969.003.0157

that it evokes, even if that response is an internal experience? From there, we can make better-informed decisions of how and with what to pair it. This also applies from thinking in the other direction: When considering your desired response, what stimuli might already "belong" to it?

Take the example of bell training to get towards an orgasm. A bell and orgasms might not appear to belong together at first. For some people, this might be a stretch: The ringing of a bell just might not be that sexy to them. Consider, though, that for others, the bell symbolizes Pavlov and training, and so it might be the perfect, nicely cliched tool. Maybe for some people this would be a dog clicker, or a snap of the fingers, or your voice saying to them, "Now." And these, of course, are just auditory stimuli. As with everything, it's key to strive to understand your partner's thought processes and responses in order to control them.

But what about the idea of using hypnosis or other tools to change how your subject feels about a certain stimulus? This is a great method and fun to "cheat" with, and is certainly fair game. If your subject thinks that bell-ringing is silly or nonsexual, you can convince them hypnotically or otherwise of the association with eroticisim, perhaps talking about how it's a classical method to train them, and training turns them on. For some, maybe this takes a different form, explaining the use of the bell as a private toy, making a special and fun trip to find one and gift to them, creating that shared feeling of intimacy. Sometimes, forcing this belongingness is very useful and a rather fun exercise all on its own, but consider that you can always do less work by going with the flow and utilizing the subject's own natural thoughts and responses.

CHAPTER 4: OPERANT CONDITIONING

Operant conditioning can be defined as: "A form of learning in which behaviors are dependent on, or controlled by its rewards and consequences."[6] As mentioned before, this is the part of conditioning that is often thought of associated with ideas like carrot and stick metaphors, clicker training, or punishment spankings. It is absolutely a useful way to intentionally train—or, to use learning language, teach—behaviors, but also looked at from a different perspective, it describes why people learn behaviors (from unintentional operant conditioning). Just like with classical conditioning, operant conditioning also factors heavily into why we do some of the things that we do in hypnosis.

Definitions

A lot of us are familiar with the terms "positive

---

[6] Shrestha, P. (2019, June 16). Operant Conditioning Definition and Concepts. Retrieved from http://www.psychestudy.com/behavioral/learning-memory/operant-conditioning/definition-concepts.

reinforcement" and "negative reinforcement," and use them to mean "rewards" and "punishments" respectively, but operant conditioning is more specific and in some places entirely contradicts the colloquial definitions with which we are familiar. In some ways, defining the vocabulary helps to define the concepts.

In the terms we use in operant conditioning:

- Positive (+): To add a stimulus
- Negative (-): To take away a stimulus
- Reinforcement (R): To encourage a behavior
- Punishment (P): To discourage a behavior

So from this we can move on and more easily understand the main processes of operant conditioning. Here, we'll explore each of the parts and offer a couple examples: One example of effective operant conditioning without hypnosis and one in which hypnosis is applied to operant conditioning.

- Positive reinforcement (+R): Behavior is encouraged by adding a favorable stimulus
    - Non-hypnotic: You ask your partner to bring you a slice of cake, and they deliver it. You smile and genuinely thank them.
    - Hypnotic: You tell your partner that their mouth feels oh-so-good on you. They feel a rush of sexual pleasure, as suggested for when you praise them.
- Negative reinforcement (-R): In behavior that has an aversive stimulus attached, that stimulus is removed so that the behavior is encouraged
    - Non-hypnotic: Your partner has heard you speak disapprovingly about their habit of cluttering their room. They clean, knowing it will stop you from saying those things,

and you cease making comments.
    - Hypnotic: While they're trying to fit something deep into their mouth, you suggest to your partner that there is no discomfort whatsoever on their throat.
- Positive punishment (+P): Behavior is discouraged by adding a stimulus that is found aversive
    - Non-hypnotic: Your partner ignores an important order. You give them a stern talking-to.
    - Hypnotic: Your partner ignores an important order. You hypnotically give them the experience of giving them a talking-to.
- Negative punishment (-P): In behavior that has a favorable stimulus attached, that stimulus is removed so that the behavior is discouraged
    - Non-hypnotic: Your partner puts off doing the laundry because they are so into playing their video game. You take away their game system.
    - Hypnotic: You want to tease and deny your partner and stop them from masturbating. You hypnotically remove the pleasure from them touching themselves.

These are at the core of intentional (and unintentional) behavior modification. The examples given to start us off are "desirable" examples of operant conditioning; that is, the conditioning is being applied effectively for good results (making some assumptions about what those are). There are also "undesirable" forms of operant conditioning, which may occur where a behavior is pushed in an unwanted direction, often from unawareness that reinforcement or punishment is occurring. For example, if your partner has been struggling with following through on an instruction to greet you a certain way, and when they do, you say something like, "It's about time you got that right," that is actually more of a positive punishment and discourages them from doing it in the future.

Reinforcement and punishment can affect behavior immediately or over time, and there are many variables that affect these processes, which we will dig into further in the chapter. However, there is one final, fundamental aspect to operant conditioning that we discussed earlier as a part of classical conditioning.

- **Extinction:** A behavior that had been previously reinforced is no longer occurring, because reinforcement has ceased.
    - Your partner gradually stops calling you by an honorific, since you stopped praising their diligence with using it.
- **Extinction bursts:** While extinction is occurring, behavior is varied (in frequency, intensity, or changed entirely) to attempt to get the same reinforcement.
    - Your partner goes through a period of calling you by an honorific nearly every sentence, sometimes even a different honorific, to try to get some reaction out of you.

The concept of extinction is a familiar one, and from some perspectives, our enemy. Oftentimes in relationships, we see the gradual decline in frequency of a behavior we like and expect but don't understand why; in some cases we assume it's laziness or indifference. In lab experiments, extinction is just the natural consequence of not reinforcing a behavior. But in relationships, extinction often means disappointment: The disappointment of the partner who expected the behavior to continue forever once learned, and the disappointment of the partner who has stopped getting the reinforcement (and oftentimes attention) they need or desire. Even in relationships where one partner can create rigid rules for another, even if the behavior for the rule is reinforced, the partner may become listless or unmotivated to uphold the rule if the "carrots," so to speak, stop being offered.

Extinction bursts also should sound familiar; many of us have had the experience where a partner will "act out" in some way in order to get attention. These are not all necessarily extinction bursts, but in some cases, certainly this can be described as them varying their behavior, sometimes emotionally, because what usually was working to give them reinforcement (attention) has ceased to give the same response. Sometimes this happens with rules or protocols that have been explicitly set up, such as in D/s relationships. But quite often this happens with behaviors that were unintentionally conditioned: The partner who grew used to your chats turning into playing every day, and if a day goes by without a scene, they become even more chatty. Unintentionally, you've associated the idea to them of talking to you with getting rewarded with play.

Things That Affect Operant Conditioning

While the main processes of operant conditioning are very simple once laid out, just like classical conditioning, there are many factors which may affect them. Let's explore some of the concepts which play a part in the effectiveness of our training.

Intent and Awareness

Something we should always keep in mind is the question, "Are my actions in line with my intent?" One of our biggest enemies in brainwashing and conditioning is not having a full grasp of what behaviors we are actually affecting, and how we are affecting them. If your partner goes out of their way to make you a nice lunch, and you are distracted and unresponsive when they give it to you, even if you say an obligatory thank you, you have given them a positive punishment. Your lack of attention is aversive, which discourages the behavior of them going out of their way for you. Of course, we are all human, and one instance of this is probably not enough for most people to become totally unmotivated, but continued, this becomes problematic. There is a marked difference between your intent (assumedly having a partner who serves you and enjoys it) and your actions (punishing when they do something that is in line with your goals).

Mixing Signals

One of the most important and complex factors to effective operant conditioning is the necessity to avoid mixing signals. As discussed previously, what is favorable to one person might be aversive to another. Even in a single partner, this might change moment to moment, depending highly on context—and in a lot of cases, perhaps a single stimulus is complicated and has facets of being both favorable and unfavorable.

There is a helpful term we use in erotic relationships called "funishment": The idea of administering something as a "punishment," but both parties actually enjoy the act and the process. It's often stated that a spanking might not be the best punishment for a masochist, but it goes further than that.

The act of telling someone not to masturbate for a week might be something they genuinely don't find favorable on one hand, but simply the attention and maybe even the idea of being denied pleasure becomes hot and attractive in its own right. Maybe they didn't even know this was something they were interested in, and maybe it's not even a conscious enjoyment. Maybe just the way that the order was given was an erotic experience for them. They don't have to be "into" the idea of orgasm denial to derive a sort of pleasure from being given an erotic punishment. Earlier we discussed the concept that for a lot of people, the fact that we are doing brainwashing, erotic behavior modification, is hot in and of itself. Logically, then, there is always the potential for your attention, even during correction, to become complicated.

We should place a high value on the idea of context. Of course a spanking can be an effective positive punishment to a masochist given the right frame of reference. In a sadomasochistic relationship, we can use spanking as an extremely deep correction, because of the intent with which it is given. Someone can be told that they are being punished and that their partner is genuinely disappointed in them.

Of course, what they experience could still be fun for them, given with a playful tone, or perhaps if they didn't understand that they had truly let their partner down. But the real sense of having disappointed someone hits very hard for a lot of people. When we are involved in relationships, we place a high value on what our partners think of us, and especially in these types of D/s ones, it is a common submissive desire to avoid displeasing the dominant. Even with "brats," who self-identify as wanting to act out (consensually) to get a rise out of their partner, have a line, usually regarding authenticity or level of emotional discomfort. That is the real positive punishment; the spanking itself may be just a formality or way to provide catharsis.

Satiation

How effective would a food reward be to a dog who just ate a full dinner? (Well, knowing some dogs, perhaps still effective...) Satiation is the concept that a reinforcement (or punishment) depends heavily on how "wanted" (or unwanted) the stimulus is at the time. Giving your partner an orgasm after they have already had 7 or 8 of them might not be the best reinforcement. (Well, knowing some partners, perhaps very good reinforcement...) Perhaps these examples serve to reinforce the point to which we keep returning: Having an understanding of your partner's wants, desires, and motivations is key to effective training and hypnosis.

Satiation also affects how often you can use a particular reinforcement over a period of time. For some people, particular reinforcements are something they become sated with very quickly, or very slowly, and very often there are other factors at play. Consider this example: Someone doing a bit of training with their partner where they carry around a little bag of chocolate chips to give them as a reward. The hotness of being reinforced very much like a dog may actually be the real reward in that situation, not the taste of the chocolate itself, which they may tire of quickly. But because they understand that they are digging into something deeper, and it is purposefully acknowledged, perhaps with some petplay elements (and all of the fun feelings that go along with that) they are able to keep it going for much longer.

Immediacy

How quickly you offer reinforcement or punishment has bearing on how effective it is. This is slightly less relevant in humans than animals, since we can often explain verbally what our response is for after the fact. However, this is still something to be aware of; while the behavior and memory of doing it are fresh in your partner's mind is a very good time to follow through on it, and the longer you wait, the less effective it may feel. Especially, for example, when the behavior is less of a "conscious" choice, such as some trance phenomena. In some ways this is about a sort of muscle memory, even mentally. The association is built far more quickly, which means faster learning.

Consistency

Consistency matters when it comes to introducing rewards and punishments. If you only reward a desired behavior at some times instead of all times, your subject will tend to learn slower or experience frustration. This also means being consistent in that you don't want to use rewards for things that don't deserve them, which is challenging to avoid.

Size

How "much" or how "big" the stimulus is can change the effectiveness of a reinforcement quite a bit. Animals and humans tend to go through a sort of process about whether or not the change is "worth" the stimulus that is given. If the reward or punishment is not perceived to be big enough, it might not be effective. If it's too big, smaller stimuli may not work to reinforce in the future. Like everything, this is enormously dependent on who, what, where, when, and why the stimulus is being given.

In "Don't Shoot the Dog," Karen Pryor asserts that with animals, the reinforcement should be "as small as you can get away with."[7] This is relevant for people as well, although what we can "get away with" is not as simple as how large the chunk of food is that we throw at them. (Usually.) There is a huge amount to consider on what someone "needs" to be a productive reinforcement. So much of this comes down to having a good understanding of your partner, and being attentive to where they are at; mood, for example, could potentially greatly affect how much reinforcement is needed for an effective change. If they're down and listless, perhaps a bigger reward is needed… or maybe for some people, even the smallest words of praise are enough to lift

---

[7] Pryor, K. (2018). *Don't Shoot the Dog!: The New Art Of Teaching and Training*. Dorking, Surrey: Ringpress Books Ltd.

their spirits. And of course, this depends on what it is, how it's given, etc. Being careful with size can help mitigate the risk of escalating too quickly.

There is another concept that Karen Pryor talks about that is the idea of a "jackpot": A reward magnitudes greater than the usual reinforcement. Taking someone out to a nice dinner for their behavior, for example, can have a tremendous effect in creating change. Consider, though, that it's important to be clear about the behaviors upon which you are acting. Pryor also mentions that jackpots can be a way to get someone to shape up quickly even before the desired behavior starts; giving someone something really nice is a great way to motivate them to act in ways to try to make you happy.

Reinforcement Schedules

Changing behavior is not as simple as always reinforcing the response every time. There are many options for "schedules of reinforcement": Frequency and consistency of reinforcement. Note that we are talking about reinforcement only here, so purely encouraging behavior, not punishment (discouraging behavior). Each of the schedules has a different effect on behavior in longevity, strength of response, and more that has been studied in laboratory and academic settings, but as we'll find, this is a simplistic view that does not take into account the intricacies in an intimate relationship. You could theoretically stick to a single schedule during the course of training, but it is usually best and more realistic to be flexible and change timing based on various factors that we will explore. These are split up into two pieces: "Continuous" schedules (all the time) and "partial" schedules (sometimes).

Continuous Reinforcement Schedule

In a continuous reinforcement schedule, reinforcement

occurs after every instance of the desired behavioral change. For example, every time your partner calls you "Master," you pat them on the head. In a continuous schedule, the tendency is to repeat the behavior as frequently as possible in order to get the reward... until the person becomes satiated with the reinforcement. It's generally best to use a continuous schedule in the early stages of learning a behavior. This makes sense, as learning tends to happen most quickly when a behavior is reinforced every time, and efficacy drops off as they grow "bored" of it.

Fixed Ratio Schedule (Partial)

In a fixed ratio schedule, the subject is given a reward after a certain, predetermined number of responses. For example, every third time that your partner calls you "Master," you pat them on the head. A fixed ratio schedule often results in a high level of responding, with bursts and lulls. Finding a good ratio has to do with factors of satiation and frequency, although since our partners are capable of human speech and understanding, they may find this schedule rigid or trite and will likely catch on quickly if you don't tell them your goal.

Variable Ratio Schedule (Partial)

In a variable ratio schedule, the subject is given a reward after a random number of responses. Randomly, after several times when your partner calls you "Master," you pat them on the head. This generally leads to reliable responses and can be good to transition to after a behavior is initially learned.

Fixed Interval Schedule (Partial)

With a fixed interval schedule, it's the amount of time between reinforcements that is taken into account. Rewards come consistently after that time interval. Approximately once per day, when your partner calls you "Master," you pat them on the head. Often, this tends to elicit a high level or response each time the subject is "expecting" the reward (consciously or unconsciously, whenever they feel they might receive it), and a dip in responsiveness just after the reward is given.

Variable Interval Schedule (Partial)

A variable interval schedule is when reinforcements are given after random time intervals. After a random amount of time, when your partner calls you "Master," you pat them on the head. This differs slightly from the variable ratio schedule in that it doesn't have to do with how many responses the subject has given, but how long it's been. Like the variable ratio schedule, this tends to be resistant to extinction and has a steady and moderate response rate.

Continuous Versus Partial

It was originally believed that using partial reinforcement schedules was the way to go to train persistent behavioral change. This makes logical sense; perhaps having instances where your partner responds to something and you don't reinforce it will get them "used to" the concept that they won't always get the reinforcement, and therefore avoid extinction and the frustration associated with extinction bursts. This is described as the "Partial Reinforcement Extinction Effect"; our friend B.F. Skinner first talked about it in his literature and it has been the subject of scrutinous study.

However, in modern field studies, this is shown to not necessarily be the universal case.[8] While partial

---

[8] Hochman, G., & Erev, I. (2013, December). The partial-reinforcement extinction effect and the contingent-sampling hypothesis. Retrieved from https://www.ncbi.nlm.nih.gov/pubmed/23595350.

reinforcement schedules tend to have a high level of responsiveness, this varies greatly according to a lot of factors, including how "attractive" the desired behavior is, or how "attractive" the alternative behavior is. Extinction still can occur, unpredicted, especially in the early stages of training.

It is easy to look at all of these options and recommendations and want to follow a steady pattern: Start with continuous reinforcement, then gradually move to partial to keep up responsiveness. The reality is that it's much more complex and subtle than this. How do you know when to change up the timing?

The more you work with your partner and understand how to see when responses are stronger and quicker, the better you will be at adapting. If your subject is getting satiated (i.e., bored, or satisfied, or uninterested with the reward), then perhaps it's best to move to something more spread out in order to keep them on their toes (or even a different reward). Maybe in some situations, they're not getting satiated, but just the opposite—it's not enough to motivate them. Perhaps you're confused why a particular behavior just won't stick, so it might be best to really continuously reinforce as much as possible to drive it in for a little while. In some cases, constantly reinforcing might be acceptable if they're not getting satiated whatsoever. They're always wanting more of that reward and are always striving to get it.

A good rule of thumb is that if you are really monitoring their responses and progress, and what you're doing is working, don't fix what isn't broken just because a study or a book told you that one is more effective than the other. It's much more relevant to consider what is going on in the present moment than to think about what works in a vacuum. If you're able to provide the reinforcement in the ways that work best for your subject, then by all means, go ahead and do that. But be prepared to change it up, either if you are getting burnt out, or the effectiveness seems to be waning. Always be attentive to both your subject and yourself.

Appreciate, Don't Neglect

Some of this might imply that in the case of partial reinforcement schedules, you want to withhold all reinforcement in some times to fit the schedule you are using. But, a simple "thank you" or show of appreciation is a reinforcement! Does this imply that we should be giving our partner the cold shoulder sometimes to ensure we're not on a continuous schedule?

Not in the slightest. Of course we want to maintain healthy and happy relationships, and nowhere in this ideal is there room for withholding affection or appreciation. If you need more logic, consider as well that the act of not giving acknowledgement—a "good pet," a "thank you"—can be easily perceived as a positive punishment; the opposite of what we want when encouraging behavior.

In some ways, this means that we are generally using some sort of continuous reinforcement schedule when we are training our partners, because in daily life we should always do things like showing them that we care and enjoy what they are doing. Think about some of the factors discussed previously such as size; for some people, a simple "thank you" is not "big enough" to effectively reinforce behavior in all circumstances. Or the idea of satiation; in a continuous schedule, the response occurs repeatedly until the subject is satiated—when does "good pet" becomes something they have had "enough" of to be satiated? This answer will be different for everyone, and different at different times.

In general, looking at these concepts academically and with a fairly clinical eye is great in terms of learning what we're actually doing in a behaviorist model, but on its own doesn't necessarily take into account what a real, healthy relationship looks like. Think of this as a guideline and a way to examine behavior by taking a step back and looking at the bigger picture, and when it comes to applying what you've learned, be comfortable with the forms of intimacy with which you're already familiar.

CHAPTER 5: SHAPING

B.F. Skinner wrote, "Operant conditioning shapes behavior as a sculptor shapes a lump of clay."[9] Shaping is an application of conditioning that refers to changing behavior incrementally, over time, towards a goal. This is done by essentially breaking the desired behavior down into small steps and reinforcing each step in the process as the subject gets further and further along. For many of our goals, this is a main approach we take in finding our successes.

For example, perhaps you want to encourage your partner to give you more blowjobs, but they're nervous about doing it. You might take the process over time, first just having them enjoy sucking on your fingers, then be near your penis or strap-on and reinforcing that (perhaps with verbal praise, or pleasure of some sort). Later, having them kiss it. And so on, until you've reached the target goal, or you change your parameters.

None of this would necessarily have to be in the same

---

[9] Skinner, B. F. (2014). Science And Human Behavior. Retrieved from www.bfskinner.org/newtestsite/wp-content/uploads/2014/02/ScienceHumanBehavior.pdf.

sexual interaction (nor should it, in most cases), but it all depends on how your partner responds. In animal training, shaping is usually done in "sessions": Concrete time blocked out for training a specific behavior and nothing else. When brainwashing our partners, we can do the same, but consider the concept that certain behaviors are something that are constantly evolving over time, every day. In this way, sessions are not relevant for these types of relationships, depending on the goal behavior. We have more to be aware of since those clear boundaries are not a factor.

Guidelines

Here are a few guidelines for effectively shaping behavior, adapted from Karen Pryor[10] and adjusted:

- Have an idea of what the target behavior is, and of each step to get there, but be flexible
    - It can be helpful, at least at first, to block your steps out and have a vague plan of how to reach the target behavior. This allows you to have a good idea if your shaping is actually a logical set of steps that can be achieved. However, be prepared to be flexible and learn as you go; perhaps the steps between are too large and need to be broken down, or they do not seem to lead reasonably to the goal.
- Ensure each step is small enough to be achievable
    - The idea with shaping is to promote success and be able to reinforce often. Large steps, while perhaps attractive in theory as potentially leading to quicker

---

[10] Pryor, K. (2000). The Ten Laws of Shaping. Retrieved from http://www.clickertraining.com/node/299.

change, tend to promote more setbacks. It is not always easy to tell how big is too big, especially with new behaviors. Repetition with little or no progress might be a sign that you have made something too hard or that something needs to be changed.
- Reinforce each step as it is learned… but after a certain period of success, raise the bar needed for reinforcement
    - Reinforcement should be given during the learning process. Once a step has been consistently mastered, challenge them to go to the next one, and be explicit in letting them know that that's how they will get the next reward. With our human partners, it's important to do this in a very positive and encouraging way; sometimes it can be jarring to suddenly stop receiving a reward (if using something explicit) for a response for which it was a consistent expectation.
- If progress goes backwards, go back over and reinforce the steps before it
    - It's normal to have fluctuations; time between training can be a factor, as well as your partner just having a particular "on" or "off" day. If you notice that steps that were previously achievable are suddenly challenging, you can start from the beginning again and "re-teach" them to reinforce again and stimulate progress.
- End the "session" (or attempt, or series of attempts) on a high note, if possible
    - You want to cultivate those moments of your partner being happy and proud of themselves, perhaps bouncing with excitement at having learned a new behavior for you. Nobody likes the feeling

of quitting something after failing; it's why we always say, "One more round!" on whatever the game of choice is when we've lost. You can fabricate these moments in some cases: If your partner failed at a certain behavior, give them an opportunity to try again. For example, if you are trying to get them to remember to call you "Master" at the end of every sentence, and they skip one, you can easily offer them the chance to succeed by prompting another sentence, and reinforce then.

A key to good brainwashing and behavior modification is being able to break down your big goals into smaller, achievable ones. To some degree, this is about understanding the goal yourself, and being able to put yourself in your partner's shoes. Learning how to view big behavioral changes as a number of small stepping stones is a skill that comes with practice and introspection.

Let Them Direct

Shaping shouldn't always be a one-sided process. Sometimes, it's your partner who will be dictating how far you go and in what direction. This might be a conscious decision they make, or something deeper. Just like how you should build an environment conducive to and encouraging them to make choices, encourage them to feel comfortable expressing what they want and be open to them taking the lead on how far they go with shaping.

As an example, consider someone who is being trained to enjoy larger sex toys. You start them slow, reinforcing this by having them occasionally using one while masturbating. But one day, they mention or ask if they can do it more. This is a great sign and an opportunity to see where they are at and then make a decision based on that—

perhaps it's time for you to transition into letting them do it whenever they feel the urge, or pushing for a higher frequency. If you're into denial, that would be a worthwhile time to tell them that they can't, and let them pine for it for a little while. Sometimes this is going to be something more spontaneous—like they start touching themselves when you are talking to or hypnotizing them. Maybe associating your voice with pleasure wasn't even necessarily one of your goals (yet). This is great, provided that it's something you both find sexy; brainwashing and shaping work best as a collaboration. It creates a sense of being personal and full of meaning.

Slow It Down

Traditionally, when we think of behavior modification, the goal is to reach the target behavior as efficiently as possible. Usually this means that we take the fewest steps and try to encourage swift change: Progress is good, right?

However, in an erotic partnership, it's sometimes worth it (and even the goal) to go purposely slow. Sometimes, it's the process that we really find hot, the idea of changing or being changed by another person. You can drag the experience out over a very long period of time to create the sense that that change is slow and powerful. Just because someone has "learned" one step of shaping doesn't mean that you have to transition to the next one. You can also purposely choose nebulous goals that don't have a real "ending" to them. In fact, most goals only have arbitrary ending conditions.

For example, you could brainwash someone into being a little more "slutty." Maybe some slutty things include sending dirty messages, taking more nude pictures of themselves, and being more flirtatious. As soon as you make any movement in any of those areas, they are already more slutty—they're being changed. You can stay on one of those for a very long time, constantly reinforcing and tweaking.

Even if it quickly becomes a learned behavior, we know that reinforcement is enjoyable and necessary, so there's no need to rush. Also, "sluttiness" is vague enough that you can always find more small behavioral changes to add on; it's simultaneously never "done" as well as never "not done."

In general, shaping doesn't have to be (and isn't, by nature) a linear process. There will always be ups and downs; times of acceleration and stagnation. This is normal, and it's best if you and your partner remember that it's not all about trying to meet a specific, expected goal as soon as possible. Take your time, be flexible, open, and curious, and enjoy the ride.

CHAPTER 6: HYPNOSIS

This book and section are not intended to teach the basics of hypnosis. At the time of this writing, there are many readily available resources from which to learn, including several that are specifically focused on the erotic side. Here you'll find some concepts that make for more effective hypnosis as well as more effective conditioning, and hopefully ways to marry the two more seamlessly. We will be discussing the use of these principles in conjunction with brainwashing, which will hopefully offer a more broad perspective on what is possible.

One More History Lesson

Before we dig into some of the tips and techniques regarding hypnosis, we should acknowledge the man from whom much of this came. Milton H. Erickson, who practiced psychotherapy and hypnosis in the 1900s, is often cited as one of the most influential people in the field. He was a maverick of sorts, pioneering a different kind of hypnotherapy than what was generally practiced at the time.

Much of his work put an emphasis on indirect language, metaphor and ambiguity, utilizing what was provided to him by his clients, and using suggestion both inside and outside of trance under the thought process that (and this is a simplification) the "unconscious mind" was always listening. In fact, his work was so renowned that he was studied and modeled along with other well-known therapists to create the basis for "Neurolinguistic Programming"—a practice that attempts to break down effective methodology for creating lasting change (see Chapter 8 for a limited discussion of selected concepts from NLP).

His model was a game-changer in the field—when so much of hypnosis was focused on the idea of putting a person into trance and then directly suggesting what they were intended to feel or experience, Erickson showed that a lot of work can be done outside of this rigid framework, and especially through the use of common, practical language. Substantial change was possible in a short amount of time (in fact, he coined the term "brief therapy"), often using the client's own worldview and responses to incite change and involve it.

Once, when asked by fellow therapists how he defined hypnosis, he replied, "It's concentrating on your own thoughts, values, memories[,] and beliefs about life."[11] This can be interpreted in many ways, but it certainly puts an emphasis on the collaborative nature of hypnosis (the hypnotist's values are just as relevant as the subject's), including how a hypnotist should use their own life experiences and model of the world to influence how they do what they do (utilizing not only the subjects' worldviews and responses, but the hypnotists' as well).

We can learn a lot from Erickson and his approach to people and hypnosis. Understanding how to apply some of

---

[11] Lankton, S. R., & Lankton, C. H. (2014). *The Answer Within: A Clinical Framework of Ericksonian Hypnotherapy.* Routledge.

his worldview to our intimate practices, especially when it comes to conditioning our partners, is incredibly valuable. After all, he was a master of changework—and what how better can we describe what we intend with brainwashing?

Plain Language

Hypnosis involves a lot of language and a lot of discussion about language. Of course, to some degree, language is very important to the practice. But perhaps word choice isn't as specific as it is made out to be. Books about Erickson, for example, sometimes seem to get bogged down in hyper-analyzing his exact style and his vernacular. While it is worthwhile to study how a master does it (and indeed, he was incredibly gifted at using metaphor and ambiguity), part of Erickson's success was due to the fact that he tranced how he talked—his "hypnotic voice" was really not very different from his conversational one.

Not everyone is a so-called conversational hypnotist, which is perfectly fine. This section is not meant to convince you that you must always speak and trance the exact same way. But what we are aiming to discuss here is the concept that we don't necessarily need to make an extraordinary effort to be precisely "hypnotic" in our speech; "normal" words can be meaningful and hypnotic.

The nature of language and conversations between people is to change each other—to get one person to think more along the lines of what the other person is thinking, whether that's to make them see another point of view, or just to understand what's going on inside their head.[12][13] Boiled down, this is hypnosis: Talking to someone has the potential to change them. If we return to learning language and conditioning, simply having a conversation is almost

---

[12] Bandler, R., & Grinder, J. (1975). *The Structure of Magic I: A Book About Language and Therapy.* Palo Alto, CA: Science and Behavior Books.
[13] Aoki, K. (1999). Introduction: Language Is a Virus. Retrieved from https://repository.law.miami.edu/umlr/vol53/iss4/21/.

always going to teach something, make some sort of an impact, or build some kind of association. Another way of looking at this is that it may be helpful not to view hypnotic inductions as about "hypnotizing" your partner or using magical language, but instead as convincing them of what you want them to believe (for example, being in trance).

We can take advantage of this in brainwashing and hypnosis as long as we recognize it, keeping it in the back of our minds: What is our partner thinking when we say a certain phrase? How is this making them feel? Are we being understood? Is this ambiguous, and how can that be interpreted? Is there an opportunity here? We don't need to use any special language patterns or tricks—in fact, it's even more urgent that we are cognizant of this when we are just speaking normally. There is something to be said for having a specific "hypnotic voice" and signalling when we are doing something intimate, but it is worthwhile to speak authentically, and to understand that doing so does not make us less hypnotic to our partners.

The Goal of Not Having a Goal

Much of what we have introduced up until now puts an emphasis on being clear and concise about why, when, and how we make changes to our partners. But, in hypnosis, especially effective hypnosis, it is key to have a model that has room for and often focuses on ambiguity as well. This may seem at odds with the goal-oriented model that has been put forth so far. But the reality is that it's quite healthy to have your goal be to not have a goal, simply tweaking and changing things to see what happens and to just discover with your partner about their reactions and responses.

In hypnosis, there is a well-loved phrase: "There is no failure; only feedback." This is often said to reinforce that what may feel like a mistake or a flub is an opportunity for learning about your partner. For example, if you are doing a scene where your goal is to have them hallucinate a teddy bear, and they mention to you that they can't see it, there is a lot to learn about them from that. Firstly, that the environment, framing, setup, and phrasing of what you offered to them wasn't producing your expected results. But there is a lot more to it than that.

There is information and opportunity in every experience we share and participate in, and more often than not, paying attention to what is there is more salient than focusing on creating something precise. Don't let your idea of a goal become the only thing you consider to be successful—relax the feeling of having specific expectations. Just because you don't get an expected response doesn't mean that it wasn't worthwhile, successful, or erotic. In fact, it is worth adopting a model which encourages every response; work to eliminate the sense that your subject can do something "wrong."

What did they experience? Were they curious about how the suggestion was going to go? Were they certain it wasn't going to work? Did they feel anything emotionally, like a sense of nostalgia when thinking about a childhood stuffed animal? Did they see something in their mind's eye, but not quite see it visually? There are many, many variables to consider here, some of which you can gain answers to through verbal feedback afterwards, by asking questions, and some of which you can read in the moment, perhaps nonverbally. Did they have any changes in affect, body language, or breathing at any moments of your setup or suggestions? Was there an opportunity for you to work with something that was already existing? And do you already have a framework for reading their nonverbal responses just by knowing them?

A Person "Can't Not Be Communicating" [14]—So Talk Back to Them

It is so important to understand that we are constantly being shaped by our environment, but it is just as important to understand that we are also constantly shaping our environment. We have reactions to everything, which even includes not having an outward reaction. We send signals to others around us about how we are feeling or thinking about something. Sometimes this is picked up consciously, such as a coworker noticing, "You look a little down today; is everything alright?" And sometimes this is unconscious, like when we get a feeling that someone is flirting with us, but we don't know why. The reality is that this is because even if we're not saying what we're feeling, our body language and nonverbal communication changes, and if we're saying what we're feeling, the content matters, but so does the tone and affect. We are always having responses, sometimes externally, and sometimes internally.

This means a lot when considering our intimate interactions. We should be conscious of what signals we are sending, and conscious of what signals our partners are sending us. Sometimes we know how our partner feels about something when we mention it to them just by looking at them and looking for any of these signs. Maybe a pursing of lips, or a movement of the eyebrows, or a slight dip of the head. Maybe there are audio cues as well, like a change in breathing or tone, or a small sound or click of the tongue. There are some generalized commonalities in nonverbal communication as well as some that we learn are specific to individuals. In conditioning, if we present an idea, reward, command, punishment, or association to our partner, we can learn a lot just by their initial unconscious reaction. We can learn how "big" a reward is to them, or

---

[14] Coates, G. (n.d.). Watzlawick's Five Axioms. Retrieved from http://www.wanterfall.com/Communication-Watzlawick's-Axioms.htm

how excited they are (or not) to have a new behavior upon which to work.

In hypnosis, understanding that your partner is always communicating is key to being effective. Sometimes the subject in a scene is going to be verbal and there is going to be more external interaction, but sometimes they will look like they are out like a light, apparently unlikely to "talk" in a traditional sense. Still, they are communicating. We can still read their reactions and respond accordingly.

Part of being a good hypnotist is becoming skilled at noticing when your subject is experiencing something. Tiny cues will say a lot, and they are often very individualized and dependent on the situation at hand, just like all hypnotic responses. Consider looking and listening more closely for these: Changes in the way their eyes move while open or under their eyelids, small noises, pupil dilation, muscle slackness, breathing shifts, even eyebrow movement—all responses that we usually acknowledge as signs of trance. Don't stop monitoring for these shifts once they are "under." We may not know exactly what a reaction means in the moment, but consider this: In human nature there is a desire to be seen, heard, and understood. So, when noticing a response, the best way for us to respond to it is by acknowledging it.

"That's Right": Yes...

One of the easiest and most effective tricks in the book is "That's right"—a staple phrase in a lot of hypnotic toolkits. But the words themselves don't really hold any magic beyond the trope of them—it's the thought process behind it.

If your subject shows a change in response, no matter how subtle, that's an opportunity for acknowledgement—and reinforcement, if it's non-negative. For example, if they are deep in trance and you are whispering softly to them, turning them on, and at a certain moment you can hear them breathe in just slightly more sharply than usual, there's your moment. Or perhaps if you notice that their eyelids go from still to fluttering. This acts as a reward, but also makes them feel like you can see into their head, the power of which absolutely cannot be overstated—it feels as though you know what they're thinking and experiencing. Not only do you learn something about what got them, but you use it to strengthen their sense of being understood. You are reacting to their reaction.

As stated, the words themselves don't really hold all the power. Similar to good conditioning, what's significant hypnotically is that you're being genuine and true to your nature. Using your own natural speech can go a long way, so instead of just saying "That's right," you could make it as simple as, "Oh yes," or "That looks good," or even just making a sound to show your appreciation and awareness of their response. Whatever you know is appropriate and authentic for your relationship with the subject. This can be very hypnotic in and of itself.

We can apply all of this to our brainwashing and our interactions with our partners, both inside and outside of hypnosis. In fact, this is just an application of operant conditioning. Creating these kinds of feedback loops is very valuable. If you are in the middle of training a behavioral change, training your own reflex to respond to your partner's responses is huge, and will create a more communicative relationship in general, no matter what form that communication takes.

"...And...": Utilization

Another familiar phrase comes from improvisational comedy—"Yes, and…" In comedy, this means that when one actor presents an idea, the other will accept it unconditionally, and then build upon it. Good improv is a great example of good communication and feedback loops, and there is a lot we can learn from it in terms of hypnosis.

We've discussed the idea of "yes-ing" at our partners extensively and the forms and functions that can take. Where does the "and-ing" come in?

Anything can be used as a tool for effective hypnosis and change. A skilled hypnotist should strive to use what is given to them by the subject and what they observe to facilitate trance and other phenomena; if their partner is sitting with legs crossed, breathing shallowly, for example, weaving that into the induction. Or if their breath catches when you look at them a certain way, digging into that and making that focal to the scene. Sometimes these come from verbal places, as well; if you notice your partner frequently bringing up a particular interest, you know to press and take advantage of that. Maybe this takes the form of some fun, sneaky language, like if a partner says to you, "I'm a little nervous, but excited about trying this…" and you reply with, "I'm sure you are; I'd probably be a little nervous too, but sometimes that can even add to how good the scenes are, right?" "Yes"—acknowledging their nerves—then "and"—using it to your advantage.

Utilization is one of the most essential tools we have. There are schools of thought in hypnosis that talk about it as the single most basic principle—reacting to a person's natural responses as the primary method of inducing trance. It is highly effective, and it can't be stressed enough that it, just like conditioning, is more than just a set of techniques—it's a mindset.

This too should be applied to our larger brainwashing practices. If we take the mindset that our partners' responses and behaviors are constructive opportunities, it provides us with more interesting and effective ways to train and associate. If you're brainwashing your partner to feel your presence and control as something persistent, pay attention to what they signal to be the most easily accessible parts of that are for them. Likewise, this is a way to creatively and spontaneously find things to condition, whether that's from noticing patterns of behavior, noticing a new behavior that your partner gets excited about, or something else. In a lot of ways, utilization is about flexibility, which is an essential skill in training.

Pulling It All Together

To some degree, hypnosis scenes, brainwashing, and relationships in general can be seen as feedback loops of communication and behavior. "Yes, and…" is more than just a single reaction and response. It is the creation of a scene, constantly building one layer on top of another, both participants communicating to make something greater than the sum of their parts. It is about both parties constantly learning how to be more inventive and adaptable in order to make an experience mutually satisfying.

Great hypnosis is collaborative and communicative. The way your partner breathes in anticipation gives you a lot of information to work with, and the way that you respond to that gives them an opportunity to have their own reaction, creating flow. If they are verbal in some form, that's another way that they're adding onto the scene. Even your silence and pauses set a rhythm and continue to build mood and tone.

It is much the same in brainwashing and conditioning. If your partner's eyes light up at a certain reinforcement (or punishment), you can follow through to your liking, and then create a meaningful interaction just in the moments of training. You can use this principle to shape how you brainwash; informing your choices of what to influence based on your partner, and then encouraging them to respond and add genuinely.

What we should take from this is that both people are always bringing something to the table, and we can train ourselves (or our subjects) to acknowledge, respond, and build off of it. This is true in every aspect of a relationship, and especially true for intimacy.

CHAPTER 7: APPLICATIONS AND CONSIDERATIONS

In this chapter, we'll be expanding on the foundations of what we've learned so far. We've outlined the basics, but now we're going to go in depth about a few things to consider when applying these techniques to brainwashing your partner, and ways that you might use them.

Choice

Beyond understanding that conditioning involves something of a mindset for both hypnotist and subject, there is another model and perspective that is very helpful for describing how we make things happen. Consider that at every turn in brainwashing and in relationships, you have choices available to you. To some degree, it is about understanding what options you have. On another hand, it's about making multiple series of decisions that lead into one another and help to continue your goals. A lot of this is about learning how to quickly evaluate what your choices are in any given circumstance.

You can think of this as a path of sorts. One choice may open up other choices. For example, if your partner is begging you to put them in trance, you have an opportunity. You could give them what they want, which allows you to reinforce their begging and creates the chance for a scene. You could deny them, and tell them to earn it, leading them to learn how to get creative with their submission and producing a fun sense of anticipation. You could tell them that they have to do something specific, building on existing training. There would of course be other options depending on the specific situation.

Sometimes, you may choose to make a decision because it feels like the best one. Other times, you may want to choose an option just to see what other choices become available. Once you begin to think in terms of choices and possibilities, you can learn how to explore and be more inventive.

Teach Choice to Your Partner

You are not the only one who has choices in your relationship. Sometimes, brainwashing is less about directly ordering your partner to behave a certain way, but trusting that if you are being productive, they will do what you want by the nature of your own behavior. This allows for a sense that it is self-directed learning, which is one of the most effective ways for a response to become persistent. This is sort of the "show, don't tell" of conditioning: Allowing your partner to come to their own conclusion that doing what you want them to do (whether they know that it was your idea or not) is the right choice.

For example, consider that your partner is coming over for a date. They have learned that you enjoy seeing them all dolled up, so without you prompting, they decide to put on makeup and a special outfit. They start to make these decisions, which happen to be in line with your tastes, just because it makes them happy to make you happy. You've taught them that making different attempts to please you is worth doing based on your responses in the past; they start making choices based on this.

People in general will tend to make what they perceive to be the best choice for themselves in any given scenario, whether consciously or unconsciously. We've discussed that if a person learns to expect a reinforcement, this may potentially affect their behavior. In a lot of ways, conditioning someone is about teaching them that they have a choice available to them that is the most attractive option—yours.

Ethics, Effectiveness, and Relationship Maintenance in Operant Conditioning

It's prudent to mention at this point that while all of the processes outlined thus far are well worth knowing and understanding so we can reflect on our behavior, practically when it comes to an erotic relationship, intentional positive reinforcement is generally the way to go. Of course, there are times when correction is needed. But mostly, it is best to not be so heavy-handed. A simple, kind verbal correction goes a long way as a positive punishment, especially if your partner is motivated to please you (something that can be brainwashed into them). We want to maintain happy, healthy relationships, and it is much easier on everyone emotionally to rely mainly on the nice things.

All of this, as well, is highly complicated by the fact that we are engaging in erotic behavior modification: Just the act of training itself can be very sexy for a lot of people. The idea that we are doing "brainwashing," the idea that any behavior might be followed by something meant to intentionally change it in one direction or another is hot! So the concept of not wanting to mix signals, while extremely relevant, becomes challenging. It is easiest to work with and assume that the enjoyable things are enjoyable; ideally, in many cases, the whole process is seen and associated with something fun and intimate. It is generally desirable for your partner to be motivated to do this with you.

With hypnosis this is especially true. Most parts of an intimate hypnotic interaction rely on positive reinforcement; we are constantly using praise in our patter, for example. A lot of this is about building positive associations with us as the hypnotists, teaching our partners that it's good and OK to let go for us, that we will take care of them, that we will make them want more. There generally isn't much place in hypnosis for punishment in general; surely there are scenes which could involve hypnotically-induced pain as a potential demotivator, but unless you are playing with someone who on some level is enjoying it sadomasochistically, it's hard to see why you would want to teach your partner that unpleasant things happen when you are intimate with them.

We have to take this even further when we are examining our approach in effective hypnosis itself. Attempting to demotivate certain responses using punishment—for example, applying the aversive stimulus of telling your partner that you don't like it when their eyes roll up in trance—has a great risk of demotivating responsiveness in general. This is a huge pitfall and there are several reasons why we can imagine this to be the case. In one way, the person is now hyper-aware of the response you dislike and may be actively trying to extinguish it all on their own. This may cause a feeling of them being "in their head" during hypnotic interactions, not focused on you or the subjective experience of "letting go" that is so attractive. There is another concept to think about, which is how free the person feels in responding to you. One of the best experiences as a hypnotic subject is having confidence that whatever they are doing, they are doing it right; in fact, this is one of the first principles taught to novice hypnotists. Why directly contradict that?

In a worst case scenario, intentionally using hypnotic punishments could be just a bad ethical decision and could harm your relationship. Fabricating unpleasant emotional states is generally a bad idea except in some mutually enjoyable sadomasochistic contexts; there is no reason to unduly put your partner under that kind of stress when it can be easily avoided. Perhaps an easy example is the idea of using a hypnotic positive punishment of making someone feel sad when they disobey. This is unnecessary—they probably already feel bad when they make a mistake, and it would be cruel to make that even more intense for them. Besides this, one of the pitfalls is that experiencing a truly negative hypnotic response has a chance of not being effective (they won't be motivated to make it happen), which will generally decrease hypnotic responsiveness and rapport in general. Ideally, we should be hyper-aware of keeping our partners healthy both physically and emotionally.

Cognitive Versus Behavioral Change

Skinner saw "private events" or internal responses such as thoughts and beliefs to be examples of behavior. While this doesn't tell the full cognitive picture by modern psychology standards, it's a decent model for learning how to condition and brainwash our partners. We can affect patterns of thinking in the same ways that we can affect behavior. Influencing cognition can be expanded upon as something that influences external behaviors on its own, and vice versa. The two are inevitably entwined, although there are some considerations to each.

For example, if you want to encourage your partner to show more initiative in their flirtatious advances towards you, that may have a lot to do with how they think about themselves or the situation. Perhaps they see being forward in that way to be a more "dominant" action, and as a submissive in the relationship, that makes them uncomfortable. In that situation, it may be about changing the way they think about flirting, and reframing it to be more attractive. Maybe it has more to do with their self-confidence and the way that they see themselves, or how they think that you see them. It could even be that they're worried about disappointing you. All of this will affect their behavior and is something on which you can work.

When it comes to changing thought patterns, there will be times when it is most observable in how they manifest through responses. We should always be asking ourselves, "What is going on inside their head that is influencing how they act or how they seem?" This could be something we want to change, like the previous examples, or be something positive that we want to encourage, like their positive perception of us, or how they feel that we control them in pleasurable ways.

One item to note is that beliefs and thoughts can often feel more automatic, impulsive, or out of one's "conscious control" than behaviors, which may feel like they require action. This has its pros and cons. On one hand, it can be frustrating for someone to try to change thought processes that they feel stuck in or don't identify with. But on the other, even when small change does happen, that can feel like proof of brainwashing, happily disconnected from their own efforts. It is worth considering that in general, it may be easier to add or change existing thoughts or patterns rather than outright removing them—think of how difficult it is to not think of something (like pink elephants, or losing The Game[15]). This is a good reason for us to remember not to punish unwanted thoughts (as they are often impulsive), but to reinforce instead (taking advantage of the impulsivity).

---

[15] The author must say that she has "lost The Game"—a mental game in which the only objective is to forget that you are playing it, and you are obligated to announce if you remember.

Persistence Versus Permanence

It is impossible to objectively view a change as permanent. Permanence implies that something will never shift again; by now, we've explored just through the limited knowledge of this book that behaviors are affected by many factors and change all the time in subtle or substantial ways. No technique, hypnotic or otherwise, can make a change magically immutable. (See Chapter 11 for discussion of "undoing" changes.)

When dealing with brainwashing, which involves cognitive and behavioral change, it is best to think in terms of persistence, instead. This allows for natural shifting—for both you and your partner to understand that if there is change, it doesn't denote failure. In fact, even when we're aiming for persistence, it's necessary to allow for some wiggle room and even to celebrate it; it can be a great tool to go with the flow of someone's patterns.

One of the best ways to make something feel as persistent as possible is instead of changing the behavior to fit the rules, change the rules to fit the behavior. For example, if you want a persistent change in the form of your partner always feeling submissive to you, you can define "submissive" very broadly—"Even a hint here and there, finding yourself thinking of me, fantasies that you don't even notice having," for example. This may overlap with behaviors they're already having, thus fitting what they already do into the "brainwashing success" category. This is something that you can do while setting up, or reinforcing a particular response that they come to you with naturally ("I've noticed that I feel xyz here and there…" "Of course you do…").

Persistence also has to do with upkeep, of course, so creating behavioral changes that are self-reinforcing is beneficial. You can alter the way that someone thinks about these changes so that they become rewarded by their own thoughts about them. Likening these patterns to "earworms" might be one way of doing this, causing someone to think or do them over and over, creating a sort of mental muscle memory for it and thus causing it to be quite persistent.

It can be fun in terms of fantasy to talk about permanent change, but also consider the concept of "temporary permanence"—times where something may feel permanent, but for a limited time. In all of these cases, it is good practice to keep your partner on the same page about all of this; there is no sense in leaving them in the dark and feeling bad if they have responses that they feel are "wrong."

The "Brainwasher" Is Also Brainwashed

"Brainwashing" is not a one-way street. The way that partners change each other and evolve over time within the context of interpersonal relationships is in some ways obvious and in other ways overlooked. We have spent a lot of time talking about how conditioning affects every person as a function of how we learn and grow, so naturally it stands to reason that even if we are all-powerful mind controlling dominants, we are not immune to this kind of change.

This can of course be advantageous—when we learn to expect behaviors and get into habits of reinforcing at the right times, when to look and pay attention, having our own positive "reward" responses when we see behavior we like, and so on. It's also worth noting that we may go through some of the same challenging experiences that our partners go through, such as feelings of dependency; we talked in Chapter 2 about how risks in this sort of play are not only risks for the bottom.

It is helpful to be aware of how we start to go through our own processes as "brainwashers" and how our behavior and cognition may change over time, whether that's based on or independent of the things that we are doing in our relationships. Perhaps we may begin to become aware of patterns that we go through and shift our own behavior to be more reactive and responsive in positive ways. After all, we have all the tools for it, and learning about how we think and behave may be an educational experience in how our partners do the same.

THE BRAINWASHING BOOK

CHAPTER 8: TOOLS

In this section, we'll be talking about some of the ways we can merge hypnosis and conditioning, effectively using one for the other and vice versa. When we think about adding hypnosis to enhance conditioning, we should start by thinking about how hypnosis adds a level of options available to us for reinforcement and punishment. We are modifying the behavior by adding or removing stimuli, not modifying the behavior directly through hypnosis. To some degree, this is about creativity and efficiency; operant and classical conditioning alone can help us to achieve many of our goals without hypnosis. So it becomes a fun process of stretching our minds and being able to incorporate hypnosis into our lives in a more tangible way, maybe even outside of traditional scenes. Using suggestion to alter factors like size and satiation of our reinforcements is another way to go about this. On the other hand, perhaps we can consider the possibility that hypnosis can provide something more effective than traditional reinforcement.

We'll also be going in-depth about some well-loved tropes and techniques to see how they apply, as well as breaking them down to further understand how to utilize them in brainwashing and hypnosis in general. Periodically revisiting the basics with a new perspective (such as our growing knowledge of conditioning and hypnosis) allows us to become more comfortable and effective with them in our practice.

Lastly, some new concepts will be introduced that may be considered intermediate or advanced discussion related to hypnosis and brainwashing. In general, this chapter is meant to be somewhat of a "catch-all" for some of the informational tools, tricks, and techniques we have available to us.

Conditioned Reinforcers

The intersections between classical and operant conditioning are many, but one of the most useful marriages of the two is the creation and use of "conditioned reinforcers." All organisms have basic drives—the need for food and water, for example. These are called primary reinforcers, because they are already present, and there is no pairing that has to happen to elicit them. A conditioned reinforcer, on the other hand, is a stimulus that's been classically trained into the subject to act as a reward for operant conditioning. An example of this would famously be a dog clicker (which of course could be relevant for dogs or kinky humans).

Conditioned reinforcers can manifest spontaneously or without conscious intent, just like any classically conditioned response. If you're frequently texting or messaging nice things with a partner, maybe seeing the icon pop up or hearing the sound of the notification gives you that good, excited feeling. It's not the sound or sight of the messenger that is the reward, but your brain is expecting the good feelings you get when talking to them, based on more foundational drives.

We can, of course, create conditioned reinforcers that

suit our needs when it comes to operant conditioning and training. Dog clickers or other objects with reliable tones are common to use for marking rewards. Even the words "Thank you" or "Very good" are already trained into us to be reinforcing. We can give them extra oomph by using hypnosis to change the kind or sense or intensity of the reward it gives, or we could do it with careful pairing and training.

Examples of conditioned reinforcers:

- "Good girl/boy/pet/toy"
- "That makes me so happy"
- Head pats
- Bell sound
- Applause

Anchoring/Triggers

"Triggers" are often one of the first concepts that hypnotists learn about. The idea of hypnotizing a person to have a certain suggested response elicited by some signal is a common desire and often an easy enough one to implement, in theory. For example, when the hypnotist snaps their fingers, the masochistic subject feels like they're being flicked with a whip. "Anchors" work on a similar concept—there is an implication of it being an emotional state that is evoked, but it could be broadened to mean, again, a behavior brought about by a signal. An example of an anchor might be that when the subject squeezes their hand into a fist, they feel happy, or maybe a little drunk.

Triggers and anchors allow us to automate some of the responses we might want our partners to experience in terms of types of reinforcements, such as praise and pleasure, which we will discuss. But, if we look at hypnosis with a critical eye, we can see that much of the foundation of "why" certain principles work has to do with operant and classical conditioning. When we bring out our shiny pocket watch and our subject smiles and blushes, that's the result of an associated response. When we say the word "drop" and our subject crumples over into trance, that too works on the same idea. Our subjects learn how to go into trance, and we praise them for their responsiveness. It is all interconnected.

Perhaps this can allow us to be more hypnotically effective—learning that simultaneous conditioning is not the most effective method of pairing responses may cause us to want to lean towards using a trigger that precedes the desired response instead of happening at the same time. And in terms of anchoring, we can understand that there are certain steps we want to take to try to avoid the response becoming extinct. We've learned about belongingness and why some things pair more easily with others, so that might influence what signal or trigger we use to elicit a feeling or behavior.

Likewise, understanding how to best utilize triggers allows us to be very creative when conditioning behavior. There is a large breadth of stimuli that can act as a positive reinforcement, beyond just straight pleasure—for example, doing something fun and performative, such as meowing like a cat for a petplay-inclined person, or getting stuck momentarily on their own thoughts, blanking out for just a moment when they do something right.

Examples of triggers:

When…

- You snap your fingers
- You touch their shoulder
- You say a specific word or phrase
- They think about you
- They put their head on their pillow
- They start to masturbate

They…

- Feel some kind of pleasure
- Get dumber
- Make a noise or say a phrase
- Forget the last five seconds
- Freeze
- Change personalities or become doll-like

Pleasure

Perhaps the most obvious utilization for many of us is the idea of hypnotically suggesting pleasure as a reinforcement. Instead of relying on physical stimulation, or simple praise, we can take advantage of the way that our partners can experience pleasure through suggestion. In a very broad definition, "pleasure" is the only application for positive reinforcement, as it assumes the subject is getting something good (pleasurable) out of the stimulus. Given the recommendation for positive reinforcement over much anything else, this is a good use, but there is a lot to consider.

Sexual Pleasure

There are many different kinds of pleasure. Sexual pleasure is the one that jumps out immediately, of course; there is something very hot about conditioning someone using their sexuality, and this falls quite in line with the trope of "brainwashing" as many of us know it. So certainly, suggesting or implementing that your partner will experience sexual pleasure when behaving in line with your goals is an option.

Not only does it tend to be more effective as we learned with the concept of "belongingness," but there is something pleasingly thematic about using a reinforcement that fits the behavior, so using sexual pleasure to encourage sexual acts might be one way of doing this. This may avoid mixing signals, if you don't necessarily want your partner to get aroused every time they complete a nonsexual task for you. But that is only one model of using it.

Sexual pleasure comes in many forms, as well; there is the feeling of arousal, the feeling of being stimulated, an orgasm, and much more. Maybe an orgasm isn't practical or possible for your partner as a reward, or maybe it is. Maybe having them experience a "mini-orgasm," or an orgasm in the part of their body that is connected to the behavior you're encouraging. There are all sorts of parts to an orgasm, too—the build up, the edge, the climax, the coming down. And for a lot of people, there are different "kinds" of orgasms.

Examples of sexual pleasure:

- Increasing the physical sensations of having your partner touch themselves
- Feeling an intense jolt of pleasure to which they can't react
- Having a vivid recollection of the best sex they've ever had
- Hitting the edge of an orgasm
- Feeling the heat of arousal spread slowly through them
- Becoming engulfed or consumed with a sense of ecstasy

Emotional Pleasure

Emotional pleasure is an underused tool. It is fun to suggest and just happiness itself can range from a little surge of something that makes you smile to total euphoria, with infinite variation in between. This becomes great to use as part of positive reinforcement; absolutely ensure that your praise hits the mark every time and is not distracting in a sexual way or inappropriate for the situation. For some subjects, responding to a suggestion exactly as the hypnotist phrases it is not as easy; depending on what is involved, manifesting an emotional state or a more abstract form of pleasure might be easier. Of course, vice versa; everyone is different.

For example, some subjects have difficulties with kinesthetic hallucinations. One way you might work on that is by suggesting that they have the emotional reaction that they usually have when the phantom touch is suggested (for example, a stroke of their hair). In this way, it is easier for them to recall what they feel emotionally when they feel you stroking their hair. A lot of the time when we are suggesting something physical, we are seeking the abstract, "mental" feelings as much as the physical ones.

Using this model of "the feeling you get when…" allows us quite a bit of variety for the types of emotional pleasure we use with our partners, and gives us some good ideas. For example, what about "the feeling you get when you kneel in front of me?" This speaks to a feeling of submission that some of our partners might experience which is certainly a type of emotional pleasure for some people. Perhaps this even reinforces a mindset that you're trying to keep as one of your brainwashing goals.

Examples of emotional pleasure:

- The feeling of winning a game
- The feeling of achieving a goal that's been set for a long time
- The feeling of pleasing their partner
- The feeling of being carefree
- The feeling of being fulfilled or satisfied
- The feeling of being a "10" on a scale of 1-10
- The feeling of being a well-loved pet
- The feeling of being under your thumb

Praise

In many respects, verbal or nonverbal praise is often thought of as the bread and butter of positive reinforcement. When a dog fetches a ball, it is almost reflexive for us to become joyful, pet them, and say (often in a high-pitched voice), "Good boy!" With our partners, this is also true (metaphorically, or down to the somewhat condescending tone and head pats, if they're into it).

Praise plays an important role in our relationships, not just in terms of brainwashing or behavior modification, but in maintaining something healthy and sustainable. Praise is telling your partner "Thank you" for making the bed, or "You look amazing today" when they clearly put in a little extra effort.

We also use praise all the time in hypnosis. The ideal is often to get to a place where your partner knows and feels praised for their responses—everything they do is right. This encourages a greater depth of responsiveness from them, not only because they feel like every response is a positive response, but because they feel seen. We can apply a similar principle outside of hypnosis; we want our partners to feel like we are seeing them, and giving praise is a way to play into that.

In the vanilla world, we often have a prescribed model of what the right kind of praise is to give based on our relationship with the person. Between a human and their dog, we rely a lot on tone and excitement as well as simple words. With a parent and child, there are different things which are appropriate to say at different age groups ("Wow, what a good job you did!" versus "I'm proud of you"). In relationships, there is often romanticism involved in how we praise our partners.

In the kink world, we have the luxury of adopting these from different authority models and using them how we see fit. This is an opportunity to experiment and get creative. It doesn't have to be puppy-play to say, "'Atta girl!" to your partner. You can build praise around your dynamics, just make sure that it's sincere. With hypnosis, of course, we can add on "extras" to our praise—maybe ensuring that it always hits home, or coupling it with some kind of trigger.

Compliments in particular can be complicated for some people. Some people may get embarrassed by praise, especially if it is highlighting an aspect of themselves about which they feel insecurity. You can work with this in different ways, whether that is conditioning them out of it ("If you get complimented, you have to say, 'Thank you'"), encouraging it as a fun humiliation game (positive reinforcement), or building an environment where they get used to being praised and enjoying it. In particular, talking about appearance can be very intense. Everyone has different "tender places," so it may be worth proceeding slowly.

As with every aspect of conditioning and brainwashing, we have to think and be conscious: What are you praising? What does your partner think you're praising? Are you on the same page with them? We always want to be very sure that we minimize mixed messages if we're not intentionally trying to be ambiguous. Praise can be about anything, but if your partner is being praised for something they aren't aware of, it has a second job, which is to highlight that accomplishment.

The most fundamental concept is that our praise isn't empty—it must come from a genuine place. Some of our partners may have preferences in how they like or don't like to be praised, and it's good to take that into account, but being true to the way that you want to speak, or the things you want to say will help keep everything feeling real and rich, and much more effective.

Examples of praise:

- "Oh yeah, that's hot"
- "You're doing so well"

- "Look how pretty your eyes are when they flutter"
- "So responsive"
- "What a good dolly"
- "Wow, you're such a dumb bimbo"

Mantras

A popular hypnotic device is the mantra: Getting a subject to verbally or nonverbally repeat a word or set of words. Mantras can be anything, from the simple "In… Out…" of breath, to something like "My mind is blank…" or even "I am a brainwashed slave." This is often for mutual arousal, but it also comes from the idea of conditioning someone to believe the phrase and its meaning, if transiently. Some mantras are of the "call and response" variety—the hypnotist says a phrase that triggers the subject to either repeat it or respond with an associated phrase. ("You are…" "…So deep…") Mantras are fun and useful and seem like a no-brainer example of both operant and classical conditioning, but there's a lot to unpack to get the most out of using them.

Mantras are sort of multi-layered in terms of what associations they build. Looking at the operant conditioning side, mantras can be great reinforcers on their own or on top of other reinforcers. It's very effective to reward your subject by allowing them the privilege of saying an erotic phrase, which may turn them on by itself or which might be already associated with pleasure. This is especially useful when we think about wanting the reward to fit the tone or task—you can customize phrases. For example, if they've done a good job making dinner for you, you can let them (or order them to) say, "I love to serve." It can be something that's said once, or repeated for a different effect. In some cases, a single instance will be very impactful, perhaps leaving them wanting more (which, as we explored, can be very positive in terms of play or delivering rewards). For some people, repetition is a powerful thing that can alter their headspace. Having gone over the idea of reinforcement schedules, it's easy to see that mantras function as other reinforcers do in respect to where we have options for introducing them.

On the other side, we can see that mantras also involve classical conditioning, and in different ways. To be an effective reinforcer for operant conditioning, the phrase should be associated with a positive response of some sort already. In some cases, this happens naturally, as repeating a mantra can be a turn-on in and of itself. It's also easy to see that over time, reusing mantras allows us to draw upon the depth of history that is built between intimate partners—very powerful. Of course, as we discussed, there is more than one pleasure response we can evoke with suggestion and recollection, and this is true for all emotional or physical responses. This is often complex, and it's by drawing on the breadth of response that we create rich experiences.

Bringing It All Together

There's another aspect of mantras that lies somewhere between these two, and one of interest to many: "You say these words, and something happens." The more they repeat, "I'm a pleasure doll," the more they feel like one. Now that we've gone over some of the nuts and bolts of classical conditioning, as well as goal-oriented brainwashing, we have a better idea of how to achieve this effectively.

To incite change in a person, mantras are most effective when the words are associated with something; that is, it is more impactful for a subject to repeat, "I'm a horny sex toy" while imagining what it's like to actually be a horny sex toy, or visualizing or seeing erotic images, or having some other kind of focus. What many people do is rely on the mantra itself to evoke these associations or imaginations, but it's prudent to help it along. We can set this up in advance with a sort of pre-talk, introducing and framing the mantra as corresponding to something: For example, "I want you to focus on the meaning of the words that you're saying—really think about and imagine all the things you might imagine while saying them." Or, we can slip words in while the subject is repeating, which can make for a very intense experience. (If they are saying "I must obey" over and over, you might double their words, repeat back to them, whisper words like "Obey me" or "Feels just right…" overlapping with them.) In an ideal situation, the mantra becomes its own reward, something that reliably evokes a response as well as provides a focal point for their thoughts. It also begins to have the qualities of an anchor, in this case—evoking a mindset or mental state.

Framing a mantra as something that will incite change is also helpful, as the intent and expectation is clearly set (and expectation plays a large role in response and change). Mantras can be used as a sort of hands-off reward, as well—you can set up boundaries of where and when your partner must say them. For example, every time they finish cleaning their room, they repeat, "I am a good pet." Or, you can have it running in their head during a task. You can also set up a ritual where the mantra and focus on brainwashing is the focal point—no other distractions. Making them take time out of their day to do something that you told them to do is an example of how introducing control will help their mindset.

Examples of mantras:

- "I can't think"
- "I am a dumb slut"
- "Obedience is pleasure"
- "Who is a good toy?" … "I am, Master"
- "This slave is brainwashed"
- "Going deep…" "…Is so easy"

Protocols and Rules

In many relationships, we set rules for ourselves and our partners. In vanilla relationships, they may take the form of things like not leaving our dirty laundry in the middle of the floor, or "You cook, and I do the dishes." This is a part of being a good partner to our significant others, and helps us achieve the very important task of setting and maintaining expectations. In kink or hypnotic relationships, especially when there are elements of dominance and submission, we may even have similar rules that follow that purpose, but with different tones, mindsets, or viewpoints.

Rules help us to directly set goals for behavior, and in many cases, setting them is how we communicate to our partners that we are expecting something specific. To some degree, these are often the "short term" goals referenced at the beginning of the book. For a common example, many of us expect to be called "Sir" or "Mistress" or some other honorific. Perhaps your partner is meant to keep their head high when they are talking to you, or there is a certain ritual they are supposed to perform before play. Rules and protocol don't necessarily imply a certain kind of reward or punishment when they are followed or broken, moreso they are an expression and agreement of what behaviors are expected between partners. They can be as frivolous or as practical as you like—every relationship will benefit from different approaches. You may also decide that there are times when you want some protocols to apply versus others, and of course being clear about that is key. Some relationships have explicit times when they are "high protocol"—that is, more are expected and they are more strictly observed.

It Takes Two

Protocols are opportunities for conditioning—operant in that we shape the behavior, and classical in that the behavior may come with some associations. Of course, it is our job to be cognizant of all of this. Making a rule or protocol isn't as simple as stating it once and expecting it to be done every time. We are also responsible for keeping an eye on it and rewarding (or correcting) as necessary.

Beyond this, sometimes it's not up to us to decide what a rule or protocol is. Sometimes, it's the bottom that comes to the top with an idea or a request. Sometimes that even takes the form of the top behaving in certain, predictable ways and following their own protocol. That's up to us to negotiate and decide: What level of participation we find to be acceptable or enjoyable—and, to see if it's an opportunity for reinforcement. For example, maybe it becomes a ritual to message or call each other to say goodnight if you're not in the same place. Perhaps your partner messages you first; your response may be expected, but it also becomes the reward, encouraging the behavior. Looking for these opportunities to be a part of the protocol is not only healthy and natural, but useful.

Flexibility

Relationships are living and breathing; always changing. Just as we should be flexible in how we play and brainwash, we should be flexible in our protocols. A rule that is set at one point may not fit later on, and that's perfectly fine. Sometimes this is obvious immediately—both parties are not really upholding or enforcing it. This can be a normal progression of a rule, although it's ideal to try to avoid your partner feeling like you're not noticing them. That is extinction, which we discussed in Chapters 3 and 4.

Flexibility isn't only significant when it comes to a protocol not fitting anymore, but for changes as well. The communication you get from your partner is valuable, for example, about how it is working for them as is. They may verbally tell you about a change they'd like to make, or maybe it's something unsaid that you're noticing. There's a time and a place for pushing them to do it your way, but sometimes it's best to compromise. It's always a good idea to be attentive. There is no hard and fast rule for when you should be more "strict"—weigh your options and try to understand how your partner is feeling and how they might react.

We always want our relationships to stay happy and fun. This means that if your partner isn't able to abide by a certain protocol for environmental reasons or something else outside of their control (including misunderstanding), that is not the time for punishment. Instead, consider rewarding them for making the right move—this will help reinforce the concept that you're both on the same team, and that they should continue to make choices that respect their well-being.

Examples of rules and protocols:

- Maintaining proper posture
- Asking permission for something they might normally have easy access to
- Wearing a certain item of clothing or accessory in certain situations
- Eye contact (making or not making)
- Taking a photo of themselves every day
- Opening doors or carrying items for you

"Gifts"

Gift-giving is a familiar and rewarding part of relationships. Many of us are well acquainted with receiving something special from a significant other and treasuring it, whether it's a piece of jewelry, an item of clothing, a kinky toy, or practical. When we give or receive items from someone important to us, we tend to assign a special meaning to them.

In some ways, we can look at non-physical things as gifts

as well. Taking someone on a date can be a gift. Some couples use sex acts as gifts. Making time for someone, in any way, is beneficial and valuable. When we add brainwashing into a relationship, if we reframe this, there are a lot of gifts in what we do.

Behavioral changes in general can be gift-like, and indeed, if we treat them as such, we can find new opportunities for intimacy. Your partner can learn to think fondly of you every time they do something that you conditioned into them. They may already have things that they do that remind them of you—you can take advantage of this and create even more intimate moments and associations.

Taken a step further, we can frame certain suggestions as gifts to our partners. We can give them anchors that they keep with them through their day, or mantras that they can say. In serious long-term relationships, we could even go as far as creating a sense of persistence and permanency, reminders of ownership and brainwashedness in thoughts or responses. Since these are imaginative, they can be creative and collaborative, and they can be wonderful options for relationships where there is a physical distance.

Examples of gifts:

- An anchor where they feel a rush of submissiveness when they touch a certain part of their body
- Hypnotically "replacing" a part of their body with something magical—or adding a phantom tail or wings
- The feeling of an invisible collar or piece of jewelry on them
- A certain mental state when they wear an item of clothing
- The very act of giving a suggestion

Denial

If your partner wants to have an orgasm and you tell them that they have to wait, it can create a very intense feeling of anticipation. For some people, the simple act of being denied something that they want can be very grounding and feel like a strong sense of control. It can increase arousal and sensitivity to stimulation, whether that's physical or psychological. Denial can also be used with activities besides orgasms or masturbation. You can deny or delay any kind of pleasurable experience, like gently telling them they have to resist trance as you swing a pocketwatch in front of their eyes. It's not for everyone, as for some people it can be frustrating (in a negative way), but for those who are into it, it can be a powerful tool.

Specific Versus Vague

In some cases, denial will promote obedience and the desire to be rewarded. In fact, you can set up situations where you tell your partner that they must act a certain way for them to get what they want. For example, you can tell them that they're not allowed to masturbate until they write you a journal entry. Or, you can be purposefully vague, and enjoy seeing how they behave to try to get you to give them what you've taken away. This kind of denial is very much like other kinds of operant conditioning, except that the subject doesn't know what behavior they have to do to get the reward.

You can use this opportunity to have them explore creatively—if they're not allowed to orgasm, they may try to entice you in different ways, perhaps by saying sexy things or by being very service oriented. You can pick and choose the behaviors you want to encourage. Consider as well that whenever you do finally allow them to orgasm, this sends a big message about what got you to change your mind—what do you want them to understand that they did that was so worth rewarding? This could, of course, be as simple as that they suffered beautifully—it doesn't have to be anything more specific than that.

Maintenance

The key with denial is maintaining a sense of interest and excitement. Some people may need a follow-through eventually, while others may love something more unending. These preferences may change over time and depending on the experience, as well. Denial, just like conditioning, requires attentiveness to your partner's state of mind. You need to throw them something stimulating here and there to keep momentum going. For example, if you've denied them the ability to get off with their favorite toy, sometimes you may want to allow them to touch or hold it while they masturbate, or even use it for small intervals of time. This shows them that you still remember and are attentive to their "suffering," and also provides some pleasurable stimulation. It also keeps the association between the toy and their pleasure going strong—over time, if it was too out of reach, they may stop responding to it because they stopped expecting that it was going to get them off.

Denial can last for varying lengths of time—sometimes five minutes is a long time, and sometimes weeks can be short. Of course, this varies based on who and what is involved, but this also largely depends on how well you both can keep everything fun and exciting. It shouldn't just be a one-way street—it should be enjoyable for both of you, and you both can show desire in different ways (and in some cases, playful frustration) to keep it all interesting. For example, if they're not allowed to perform oral sex on you, you both may be expressing a want for each other, which may lead to some hot "You can't touch me" scenes.

Watch for signs that your partner is getting too frustrated or losing interest. If they no longer seem to be trying to please you, or if they are sulking and generally seem upset, you may want to reevaluate what's going on. It may be as simple as "renewing" the denial in some way, like teasing them, or giving them a small version of what you've taken away. Or, you may need to give them what they want and start with a clean slate.

Examples of denial:

- Allowing them or instructing them to masturbate, but not orgasm—"edging"
- Total denial—no sexual pleasure
- Not allowed to moan or make sounds
- Only allowing them to orgasm under specific circumstances, like when they are giving you oral sex
- Not allowed to eat one of their favorite foods
- Not allowing them to go into trance to a beloved crystal

Causality ("Cause and Effect" and "Complex Equivalence")

While Neurolinguistic Programming (or NLP) is divisive and ill-defined in many ways, there is knowledge to glean from various aspects of it. NLP attempts to create a model for modeling people as well as specifically looking at the work of renowned therapists (including Milton Erickson) to see exactly what they were doing that was so effective. This book is not going to dive into the vast majority of NLP (although you are encouraged to do so on your own), but will address two concepts from it that are quite useful: "Cause and Effect" and "Complex Equivalence." Both of these are part of a larger attempt to break down patterns of thought and speech. From one perspective, these describe flawed ways of thinking, but from another, they are a way to induce trance or change minds.

Cause and effect patterns can be defined as "Statements implying that a particular action causes a specific reaction."[16] An example of this might be thinking, "They lowered their voice because they are hypnotizing me." Complex equivalence patterns are related; they "[suggest] that one thing is related to and means something else."[17] For example, "Being brainwashed means that I'm easily suggestible." Note that language concepts like "because," "therefore," "if/then," "this means," and other words and phrases that serve to connect and imply correlation or causality are important in both cases. NLP aims to challenge these patterns when they are problematic ("They aren't talking to me; they must dislike me") but also aims to use them as tools to create change ("You're listening really attentively, so you're probably going to go into trance much more deeply.") While the former (called the "Meta Model" in NLP) is worthwhile to research, it's the latter (the "Milton Model") that we are going to focus on here.

On the surface, these concepts appear useful for tricky language patterns, and that is true. Using them in simple suggestions is good practice. But more than just crafting single phrases with them, you should strive to understand that you can create causality as an essential element of your hypnosis, conditioning, and brainwashing as a whole. For example, if you are thinking about how you want your partner to feel controlled, orient yourself to think about why they would feel that way; how can you explain to them that this is an effect created by a cause? Is it that they are following suggestions and responding perfectly? Is it that you have implemented changes in their life? And always

---

[16] Bandler, R. (2008). *Guide to Trance-formation: How to Harness the Power of Hypnosis to Ignite Effortless and Lasting Change*. Deerfield Beach, FL: Health Communications, Inc.

[17] Bandler, R. (2008). *Guide to Trance-formation: How to Harness the Power of Hypnosis to Ignite Effortless and Lasting Change*. Deerfield Beach, FL: Health Communications, Inc.

consider the inverse: Are they doing all of these things because they are being controlled? How can you best express this to them?

One of the most simple patterns of hypnosis works adjacently to these concepts: State a few things that are already true (such as that you are observing the way their body is positioned, that they are listening to you, and that you are giving them your full attention) and follow up with suggestions (such as that you are watching their breathing slow down, or that you can see other signs of trance). This is another example of creating complex equivalence; because you are clearly pointing out truths, there is an assumption that those truths lead to or mean something else. Your partner is motivated by the initial "Yes, that's true" response that they experience, and thus the suggestive part feels like it is equated to or caused by it. It is presupposed—in reality, any part of a causality statement could potentially be vague and unverifiable. Of course, it's best to be convincing about these suggestions—the more you stretch, the more of a chance that they will do their internal check and find a disconnect.

To some degree, utilizing these principles most effectively is a result of being able to think outside of the box and see equivalence and causality in places that you might otherwise overlook. It is a mindset change, just like conditioning; where can you see these patterns in their behavior and life, and then how can you take the next step? A brainwashed person may even be more inclined to create that equivalence or causality in their own minds about what you do, and you can reinforce that way of thinking.

Examples of causality:

- You are brainwashing them because they deserve it for being so good
- Experiencing things this intensely means that they are giving up so much of their control to you

- Being this conditioned probably means that their orgasms will get stronger when they think of you
- They are going to get really good at pleasing you sexually because they have been thinking about you so much
- Absentmindedly forgetting something might mean that they are actually getting a little dumber
- Your ability to learn through conditioning makes you well-suited to being brainwashed

"Traps"

Consider the idea that to be most effective in brainwashing, we want to utilize as much "space" as possible. We want to take away the feeling that there are behaviors and patterns that do not fit within our bounds and definition of "being brainwashed." Note that the word "utilize" comes up—indeed, this is an application of utilization. In essence, the best way to make brainwashing feel all-encompassing and inescapable is to broaden the scope of the brainwashing itself; move the goalposts and rig the system rather than push your partner to jump higher. This in and of itself can be thought of as a way of convincing and teaching your partner that no matter what response they have, they are doing the right thing and being brainwashed. Essentially, make it so there are fewer and fewer ways to "fail."

For example, if you want to give your partner a mantra to repeat automatically, you may have an urge to be strict about how they say it, when they say it, or how you want it to make them feel. While this is one option, consider that actually by being more flexible, you get more broad control. Instead of being required at specific times or being said aloud, what if it had power every time it popped into their head? Or, instead of needing to make them horny, what if you made the scope of the successful brainwashing condition something even more simple and common, like having any response to it whatsoever? Another, well-known hypnotic example of this is when playful resistance is involved; making the resistance itself something that hypnotizes them. The behavior they're performing that did not fit your model of success is integrated as a reinforcement and hijacked.

This entire idea in general is essentially just an extrapolation from good hypnosis practice; we want it to feel like there are as many success conditions as possible in all of our trances. This promotes responsiveness in general and a feeling for our partners that they are always doing the right thing. As hypnotists, this is a way we can make our language and our trances inclusive to a point that most or even every response is one that furthers our goals and makes our partners feel like what they are doing is accounted for and (in amenable relationships) is controlling them. You can conceptualize this as "trapping" them, if you so choose—corrupting options that allow a non-positive response. This is useful not only within the context of conditioning, but general hypnosis, and as mentioned, draws heavily from utilization. In order to be most effective with this, you must first learn how to understand their potential responses. Notice as well that this concept may take heavily from causality.

Examples of "traps":

- They are being brainwashed even when they're processing it unconsciously and not actively thinking about it
- Even when they're not masturbating about you, it just makes the next time they do it stronger
- Going through their normal daily routines brainwashes them because they are training themselves to know how to behave well
- Both familiar and unfamiliar trance responses make them learn more about themselves as a subject and

- thus make them more suggestible
- Un-learning a behavior is just an opportunity to re-learn it and get more brainwashed
- Every time they think about you or being obedient to you, they have some sort of response, even if they're not noticing it

Control

One of the most alluring parts of a brainwashing relationship is the concept of having control over another person. It can often feel like release to the subject; having someone place restrictions on how they act or think allows them a greater sense of freedom in who they are. In fact, just like with other aspects of brainwashing, giving up control is a natural part of vanilla relationships. In the traditional progression, we slowly share finances, relax the way that we make decisions, and depend on each other, entangling our lives.

But just like the idea of brainwashing itself, how that control manifests or how you wish to implement it may vary. All of the tools we have discussed thus far in the book are ways to exert control over your partner. That may be tangible in and of itself, but there are some techniques and ideas you can be thinking about to make that sense even more broad and palpable.

Control is innately about one partner having power over the other, and directing, in various ways, how they think or behave. In a brainwashing relationship, we could say that it is happening all the time, at least all the time that the person is brainwashed; their behaviors (including their thoughts) are being influenced. But of course there are times when it may feel more intense than others; for example, when we are doing hypnosis or applying reinforcement.

For it to be as tangible as possible, one of the most simple things we can do is point it out when it's happening and reinforce it. This may serve to further the goal of our brainwashing feeling like a 24/7 experience if we are using this as a reminder. For example, you can easily shift the tone of just putting your partner into trance by using language that implies that you're directing the experience: "You're going into trance right now for me; because I'm choosing it, because I want it, because I'm controlling this."

In the same way, your partner following rules or protocols or even behavioral changes benefits from this. It keeps these elements of the relationship feeling fresh and exciting. We can easily get into ruts sometimes even when behavior is totally altered or many rules are being strictly followed. Mentioning here and there that your partner is doing what they're doing because you control it acts as reinforcement and reward. You may consider the concept that control in some ways is about your partner feeling like they do or don't have permission to do something, and in other ways, you can alter that to manifest itself as that they don't even consider other possibilities.

One partner having control may also imply that the other partner has a lack of it. Indeed, taking away, or, more accurately, replacing behaviors or thoughts is a very powerful way to frame this. Reminding someone how they used to act or very purposefully choosing to change something small but integral to how they view themselves can be very intense. This doesn't have to be huge or life changing; it could be as simple as switching their preference in underwear, what their favorite color of lipstick is, or how they wash their hands. Even the smallest and most innocuous behaviors can feel like they are "corrupted." Of course, be communicative and tread lightly.

As we've discussed, thoughts and cognitive behavior are important parts of conditioning as well. Control over these areas can be particularly intense. Orienting someone to think about you more, for example, at a certain time of day or in a certain place can touch on the feeling of mind control, which for many is a deep fantasy. This also can be simple and yet insidious; waking up and thinking of someone is both easy to set up and reinforce. This can take the form of something specific like a mantra or it can be more open-ended, like directing someone to fantasize. It doesn't have to be exclusive, either; as discussed with "trapping," you can hijack your partner's normal thought processes and include their usual functioning as a way that you exert control and create persistence.

Examples of control:

- Changing the way they respond hypnotically, like making their eye flutters more pronounced
- Telling them to dress a certain way
- Making them learn how to get better at cooking
- Only allowing them to touch a part of their body when they've asked permission
- Implanting thought patterns that they periodically get stuck in

CHAPTER 9: FANTASIES AND SCENES

As we've discussed at length, brainwashing is not a one-and-done event. It takes time, patience, and most of all, upkeep to maintain a sense of having "been brainwashed." However, the fantasy of brainwashing often goes something like this: A person is taken in for some sort of processing, they are changed and altered through some means of mind control or hypnosis, and then, climactically, they are "done"—permanently. There is a moment where they feel, "I'm brainwashed," and the process is complete.

By now, we understand that this is not how the human mind works in terms of practical change. But this fantasy often features prominently in our minds and the minds of our partners, whether it takes the form of something long-term or a simple scene. In this chapter, we'll discuss how to build scenes that allow us to both be effective as well as touch on some of these desires.

Anatomy of a Brainwashing Scene

A scene generally follows a certain form: Build up to a

climax and then some amount of cooldown. A good scene has many of these contained in one; many build ups, many small apex moments, and the contrast of slowing down here and there to create space. Take an example of a hypnosis scene: You turn to face your partner, taking their hand in yours and looking purposefully into their eyes. Their focus shifts and becomes more intense on you; maybe you draw little circles on their palm, and you can clearly see the signs of trance on their face (slackening jaw, eye or eyelid motion). You can almost feel the sense of hypnosis overcoming them in such an intimate moment, and when their eyes start fluttering just right, or you see them on the edge, you tug gently on their hand, and their head lolls forward and their eyes roll and shut.

What we would sometimes term as "just the induction" is a climactic moment in and of itself (and indeed, many of us fetishize just this)—this scene is complete, but could easily lead on to something more. Perhaps the next apex is having them get a sense of going profoundly deep, and the next is build up of arousal into orgasm. There are all sorts of climactic moments that we can manufacture, often by reading our partners and getting a good sense of their internal timing and working creatively with that.

One such climactic moment is what we've mentioned at the beginning of the chapter—the "I'm brainwashed" realization. It's wonderfully fun to have scenes that lead to this, whether it's a roleplay scenario of your partner being maligned by the "bad guy," or something more realistic where they realize just how under your control they really are. Maybe it is elaborate and they are tied to a chair, forced to watch a spinning spiral, or maybe it is much more subtle, like the powerful touch of your finger to the middle of their forehead.

Fantasy Ideas

If we extrapolate from the model of a scene, it's just a

matter of finding themes and ideas which fit into our idea of eroticism. Of course, this is a great opportunity to discuss with your partner about your mutual desires, as well as brainstorming together. Or, you can come up with ideas on your own to surprise them (within mutually acceptable boundaries). Inspiration can come from anywhere—books, TV, movies; erotica and porn; even taking cues from reality can work. They can be as planned and scripted or as spontaneous as you like. In this section, we'll go through some ideas to hopefully get the creative juices flowing. These elements are completely arbitrary and for examples only—certainly you can mix and match and alter to you and your partners' desires.

Situational Versus Tonal

There are a lot of different ways to approach scenes, but one example of how to think about them might be considering two concepts: The situation you'd like to create and the tone you'd like it to have. The situation might include some sort of roleplay scenario, or be the position that you and your partner are in; essentially, where you are, who you are, and what's going on. The tone, on the other hand, is what feelings and moods are evoked.

These are just arbitrary starting points, and exist on an infinite gradient and scale. One can lead to the other—oftentimes, if you think of one of these aspects, an idea or even many possibilities for the other will come to mind.

Example situations:

- Becoming recruited to be a member of a sexy brainwashing cult or hivemind
- Volunteering to be a test subject for a mind control ray experiment
- Going throughout their day while unknowingly being subject to subliminal messaging

- A stranger drugs their drink with something that makes them malleable or lowers their IQ
- Taken for an examination by a perverted doctor with drugs that make them docile and obedient
- A supervillain caught in the clutches of the hero with mind-bending powers
- A dolly or android brought to life and controlled by its maker
- Trapped in a room filled with spiral screens or wearing special headphones, unaware of how they got there
- Meeting for the first time as someone totally new to hypnosis
- Becoming a servant to the master of the house

All of these have different elements to them that can be broken down much further. Some of them have themes of resistance, or amnesia, or bring certain props to mind that might be used. Maybe the environment for one is vastly different than another. Who are you to them in some of these examples? Could you be someone else? Could they?

And then, of course, there is the question of what tone might be brought up.

Example tones:

- Caring and loving
- Dark and dangerous
- Devotional and exalting
- Predator and prey
- Forceful and pushing
- Playful and frisky
- Scary and chilling
- Seductive and captivating
- Authoritative and domineering

Tones have the quality of being nebulous, dynamic, and on a spectrum; that's part of what makes them interesting to consider. Staying with one situation and shifting the tone can drastically change the experience for both you and your partner. Maybe thinking about a certain mood brings ideas to mind, or vice versa—oftentimes there is a gut sense of what it might feel like, emotionally, or what might fit for you or your partner.

The Role of Creativity and Expression

To a large degree, creativity is significant in hypnosis and brainwashing. Creativity is about seeing heretofore unseen patterns, creating links between ideas, and producing or making something. In hypnosis in general and especially brainwashing, creativity is a driving force; we are looking for patterns in both ourselves and others that we can address in some way, whether that is interrupting them or encouraging them; we are striving to form associations and connections in our own minds and others' that further our mutual goals; we create profound and unique experiences and memories.

Scenes are largely about a demonstration of this. We may think that "creativity" in scenes is about what ideas we come up with, but it is more expansive than that. Having a creative scene necessitates an openness to the expression of both partners and an alertness to patterns and potential links. This takes the concept of utilization a little further and turns it more personal: We are not only using our experiences and the experiences of our partners because it is good practice, but because of a larger drive to communicate something about ourselves and be a good "listener" to others.

Take an example of a scene where you are transforming your partner into a bubbly cheerleader. However they interpret this, they will display unique and interesting behaviors: Perhaps you notice that they are saying "um" a lot—did they get a little dumb? This is your partner expressing something about their process, and it's an implicit invitation (assuming this style of play is pre-negotiated) for you to get creative and express something about yourself back at them, like an encouraging suggestion.

Negotiation and Going With the Flow

Every person and relationship is different in terms of their needs for their expectations, and figuring out where you and your partner lie is the first step. Some people need in-depth discussion of possibilities and plans to be comfortable with a scene, while others are most at ease just having their safewords and letting their partner go. It doesn't matter what your power dynamic or role is—the key is finding an approach that works equally for both parties. Over time, this may change in either direction—that's perfectly fine, and is a great example of why frequent communication is key to a healthy relationship.

It's one thing to plan out an elaborate fantasy scene and another to enact it. Much more important than sticking to the script is observing your partner and feeling everything out to the best of your ability and doing what fits from there. Sometimes scenes go exactly as you expect them to go, but a lot of the time you have to throw away your careful plan. Anyone can express a desire or need for change within a scene, and sometimes that means stopping or adjusting to something less encompassing or intense. This is often referred to as "negotiating downwards"—i.e., asking for change in the direction of lessening play, but some relationships are OK with negotiating "sideways" or even "up" during scenes—asking for different or more, although this can increase risk.

It's not a failure if you can't follow through a scene the way you planned, and it's also not always because someone is having difficulty with an aspect of it. It might be because there's a small part that no one even thought about that suddenly was amazing or hot. Taking advantage of those kinds of positive moments will make your scenes really,

really good.

Being open to change and flow allows you to adapt to what's happening and change both situation and tone as the scene itself shifts and evolves. This might mean that there are a bunch of mini-scenes in one, stories and roles being nested inside of each other, fractionating between emotional states and tones. Sometimes it might be just a natural sense of flow and evolution, or something like the progression of a narrative. As we discussed, some really good scenes are just like stories—they have the ups and downs, struggles and successes, and powerful climactic moments.

Metaphor and Creating Change From Fantasy

Even in complete fantasy scenes, there are opportunities to create real change. You can add elements of yourself and your relationship with them, relying on allegory for them to pick up. Oftentimes, the feelings will carry through roleplay, at the very least staying close to the surface and becoming easy to touch again. For example, if you create a scenario where they are a helpless and mindlessly obedient servant, this can become metaphorical, and you can take advantage of the "realness" of the sense of wanting to serve to turn it into actual behavioral change.

Metaphor is a key part of storytelling, whether it's cinematic, written, or something we use in speech to try to communicate. Metaphor is a way of creating presumed equivalence between seemingly unrelated ideas—for example, a simple metaphor may be saying something like, "Your smile brightens the room" to express how you feel about someone.

But metaphors are more than the short sentences we learned in English class. They are an essential tool when used in a more dynamic, allegorical way. Milton Erickson, who we discussed in Chapter 6, was known for using metaphor in his hypnotherapy as a way to indirectly coach clients into seeing capabilities and opportunities that they may not have seen before. Famously, he told a story about tomato plants to a chronically ill patient to illustrate the same level of attention involved between caring for a plant and managing illness.[18] A metaphor that that extends over an entire narrative like this can be called a "dynamic metaphor"[19]—it shifts and serves to tell a story. This can often involve symbolism of some sort; for another example, consider "The Lord Of The Flies," which is a well-known allegory of society involving characters who symbolize various aspects of humanity.

We use metaphors all the time in our daily speech, but as Erickson noted, they're a powerful hypnotic tool. They can be used to indirectly suggest trance or other responses (in fact, you may do this already without words by slowing down or lowering your voice while you hypnotize someone), but they can also be used in brainwashing scenes to create change. A scenario where you transform your partner into an unwitting psychology test subject getting brainwashed could be allegorical to their current situation if you have a brainwashing relationship, and it probably hits pretty close to home. Teacher/student roleplay could reinforce an existing sexy power imbalance. You could even do something more abstract, like moon and tide imagery to symbolize control. When a hypnotic subject is given a sufficiently ambiguous metaphor, it causes them to unconsciously initiate a transderivational search—they look inward to attempt to create connections and identify with some part of what the hypnotist is saying. This is a good frame of mind to facilitate change or trance.

---

[18] Roffman, A. E. (2008). Men are Grass: Bateson, Erickson, Utilization and Metaphor. *American Journal of Clinical Hypnosis*, 50(3). doi: 10.1080/00029157.2008.10401627

[19] Sijll, J. V. (n.d.). Cinematic Storytelling: Dynamic Metaphors. Retrieved from http://www.writersstore.com/cinematic-storytelling-dynamic-metaphors/.

Sometimes, this may also be as simple as having them recall the state of mind or temporary behavioral change they experienced, whether it's a simple nod or a call-back to another session. The more you draw upon states of mind or behaviors, even during roleplay or hypnosis, the more they will tend to be reinforced. Using scenes as a way of shaping—those small steps to larger goals—can also be very effective.

This also means that we need to be a little careful when enacting fantasies that we don't necessarily want to spill over, especially if we've taken advantage of it in the past. Some people are very good at separating the two, but for others, the line is more blurred, and it's not always going to be predictable. It isn't bad either way, it's just a matter of learning how your partner processes and working with them, and possibly working to teach them how to do one or the other through practice.

CHAPTER 10: RISKY, RISKIER, RISKIEST

At this point, we've explored quite a bit about behavior modification, conditioning, and hypnotic tools. This covers a lot of what "brainwashing" is, but there is an aspect upon which we have not yet fully touched. For some of us, "brainwashing" has a bit of darkness to it: A real sense of helplessness, or addiction, or other generally "evil" stuff—stuff you may not expect to find in a normal or healthy relationship. In this chapter, we'll get into some of the "what," "why not," and "how."

Even if you feel that you aren't interested in doing anything particularly dark, this chapter discusses a lot about risk mitigation and how to see risk in places you may not expect it. As we know by now, brainwashing is an inherently risky activity all on its own, and learning how to assess and reduce it is key to a healthy relationship.

What Is Riskier?

Some examples of this kind of riskier play include but are not limited to: Intentional dependency, obsession, control of emotion, addiction, and lowering the threshold of resistance. While they may be attractive, in all of these cases, consider the potential worst-case scenarios: They become hindering to healthy life and processing, they promote an inability to function independently, they create opportunities where the subject loses agency in such a way that they end up doing something that causes them (or others) some kind of harm.

When considering whether or not to add an element to your brainwashing and while it is active in play, always be asking yourself: What could go wrong? What conditions make this more or less likely? What can I do to mitigate this risk? What could I do if something goes too far? A key part of being able to manage risk is assessing it. This applies to everything we do in brainwashing; after all, risk is inherent in this kind of play, which we've discussed. This is especially salient when we start to delve into darker themes.

It is impossible to predict if or when something will go in an unexpected or negative direction. Even with the utmost care, an experience may take a bad turn. However, the key to risk mitigation is being observant, flexible, communicative, and careful.

"Risk Awareness" Means Assessment and Acceptance

In Chapter 2, we briefly discussed the idea of "RACK"—"Risk-Aware Consensual Kink"—as a model for assessing and dealing with risk in kink. Risk awareness is a necessary part of this kind of play, but it means something beyond simple understanding and mitigation.

Risk awareness also means risk acceptance. When consenting to a type of play, all parties involved absolutely must understand the risks associated with it, and then they must accept them as a possibility. For a BDSM example, someone bottoming for a rope suspension that carries a high risk of radial nerve injury ("wrist drop"—inability to properly use a hand either temporarily or permanently) may be more willing to accept that risk if their job doesn't require high technical use of their hands. Someone who is a writer may decide that the risk is too high—or they may figure that they can dictate what they're writing verbally if worst comes to worst.

For a brainwashing example, playing with addiction may be lower-risk if you and your partner live together or are otherwise able to be in fairly frequent communication. It may be more acceptable if the subject has other support mechanisms to rely on when you aren't available or has demonstrated strong self-reliance in the past. It may be less acceptable if the subject is alone or tends to have difficulty not relying on others.

However, the key in all of these scenarios is that the risk is assessed and considered as a serious possibility. There is planning and thinking ahead and open communication between partners. If the worst case or other bad scenarios are possible-to-likely and this is unacceptable or there is no way to handle it, the play should not be attempted unless that significantly changes.

Know the Rules Before You Break Them

It cannot be stressed enough that this is not starter material. There are some common safety protocols in hypnosis play in general and in brainwashing that we have discussed earlier. This type of play may seem to directly contradict some of them.

However, it's important to know and practice these principles for some time before attempting to subvert them, not only knowing the rules intellectually but knowing them internally and having them be an intimate part of your play. This allows for a logistical fallback and a muscle memory for something safer if need be.

For a prominent example, consider the concept of reducing resistance in some fashion. It should be well-known that with practice, subjects are able to ignore and take control of unwanted hypnotic suggestions. This is often something that needs to be learned and encouraged; it's not a given. Teaching your partner that they are allowed to and able to say "no" bolsters their independence and safety in a huge way, and is an extremely integral part of a healthy relationship as well as being an excellent hypnotic subject.

Before any effort is made to create the sense that they have less resistance towards you or your suggestions, they should be solidly comfortable with their sense of agency and ability to reject undesirable effects, and you should be comfortable with that as well. In an ideal situation, you should both be able to rely on that being a failsafe (and you may frame it as such) even if on some level you begin to play with teaching a sense of helplessness.

Contingency/Mitigation

There are different ways to approach any of these aspects of play, some arguably safer than others in different situations. Continuing the above example, perhaps it is less risky if you set up the lack of resistance in such a way that it extends the subject's ability to take care of themselves: Framing it as being unable to resist their own agency, your power over them becoming an assurance that they will speak up or resist if the need arises. Another option may be that you approach helplessness on a surface level while instilling a deeper sense of the ability to reject something unwanted.

There is no single best way of mitigating risk in any scenario, and the effectiveness depends largely on the situation and the people involved. It is usually best to err on the side of caution at first, and, if desired, slowly add in riskier or unfamiliar elements and assess from there. This is an opportunity to get creative with safety and framing; as with the previous examples, there are many ways that you might go about this.

Always remember that safety suggestions are a good idea, especially in terms of communicating to your partner that certain behavior (such as coming out of trance when necessary) is welcomed, but they are not infallible. Suggestions are not magical. The most effective method is often to be thorough and remember that to some degree, suggestions are about communication and follow-up more than a combination of special words said in a special state. Likewise, safety and risk mitigation are often about promoting healthy behavioral patterns in addition to permission to resist (such as rejecting unwanted suggestions).

For example, "You will find yourself addicted to me but still able to preserve your independence" is a good statement of intent, but on its own as a suggestion may not be the most exhaustive method of mitigation. As we have come to understand through learning about conditioning, we are able to influence our partners' patterns of behavior, and we want to express reinforcement when we see or experience them being self-sufficient or having agency.

To some degree, this is reliant on how well we are able to observe someone else's situation and behaviors. For this reason, if our view is blocked by distance and/or lack of consistent communication, it makes playing with all of this on a whole much riskier.

Specifics

In this section, we'll address a couple specific examples of darker play and discuss a little bit of the "how" as well as ways to mitigate risk. Both of these topics are extensive beyond what is written here; an entire book could be written about each of them, so keep in mind that they are not exhaustive. Please note as a content warning that there will be discussion of these elements within abusive relationships as well as outside of them.

Gaslighting

"Gaslighting" is a type of psychological manipulation that makes the victim put their own beliefs into question. It can be found in many different types of interactions, but is most known for being a tactic used in unhealthy romantic relationships. It involves denying the victim's feelings and perceptions, mislabelling and miscategorizing events, calling memories into question, and causing confusion. An example of this might be one partner insisting to the other, "I didn't come home late last night; you must be misremembering things. I bet you were just tired. You always blow things out of proportion when you're tired." One of the most risky aspects of this is that if used consistently, the person will get into the habit of questioning their own perception of reality and their memories. This can be psychologically damaging in excess and create undesirable reliance and unmanageable dependency.

Certainly, this sort of tactic is often used unethically and is a staple of unhealthy relationships. However, there are ways to take advantage of these concepts in a playful way for consensual fun. It can be very intense for your partner to flounder for reality, or second-guess themselves about their memories or motivations. You can add in bits of gaslighting as a flirtatious flavor, whether they're intended to be tongue-in-cheek or genuine—for example, you may want to exert power by insisting that they actually suggested your favorite food for dinner.

The core concept of gaslighting is, in essence, taking steps towards having your partner trust your words more than their own internal thought processes. This involves conditioning—rewarding them when they seem to be questioning what they believe. You can see this in moments of hesitation and take advantage of that, and purposefully create uncertainty through your words and actions.

Gaslighting is often responsive or reactionary—it's

harder to do in a vacuum or without bouncing off of someone's existing perceptions through speech. If you're looking for opportunities to use it, remember these principles:

- Denial
    - Take what they say and insist that they are remembering it wrong or thinking about it wrong. "What are you talking about? You never said that."
- Trivializing
    - Question the importance of whatever they are saying. "Is this really that big of a deal?"
- Diversion
    - Move the subject of the conversation. "Are you questioning my memory about this?"
- Telling untruths
    - Think about what makes the most suggestive or believable lie. "Are you sure you weren't going into trance then, even a little?"

Mitigation

Anything that creates dependency is going to be riskier than usual, but having an awareness of that as well as monitoring the situation to make sure it stays within mutually acceptable bounds will help.

Some examples of mitigation, in this case, have a lot to do with clarity of communication. First and foremost, as with any kind of play, you want your partner to be as informed as possible about how gaslighting works and how to recognize it. This turns it into a consensual experience and gives them more of an "out" if they need one. You should also have limits of what and when you're able to do this—for some people, it may only be appropriate during play sessions, but for others it may be on the table all the time (and anywhere in between). Some topics may be off limits, or you may do an opt-in model instead ("We can only play with gaslighting in the context of hypnosis").

With gaslighting, just as with hypnosis, there tends to be value in signalling—somehow showing that you are doing something out of the ordinary. When we do hypnosis, we often shift our affect somehow, whether it's a change in tone of voice, or a look, speech patterns, body language, etc. Exaggerating this at first until your partner learns how to pick up on these changes can be very helpful, especially in cases of playing with a tool that has higher potential for abuse. This helps your partner know when you are trying to be playful, and allows for a greater understanding and calibration of these times versus non-play times.

Addiction

Playing with the concept of addiction or obsession within a relationship is a somewhat popular trope; it can be seen as an extension of other fantasies, like having some sort of mind-altered thrall or servant. It can be very hot, but understandably has a large potential for issues.

What does it mean to be addicted or obsessed with a person? If we think about the concept of addiction in general, the idea of a drug high might come to mind. There is the sense of wanting to come back for more, and maybe dependency or the feeling that they can't help themselves. Indulgence is a key part of addiction—the act of engaging with the object of addiction is relieving, pleasurable, and perhaps even feels a little bit transgressive.

Being addicted to a person may not be such an unfamiliar feeling—many of us have the experience of having had a very intense crush, or first love, where we just couldn't get enough of someone's company. We thought spending time with them was the most amazing thing in the world. Everything they said was smart and funny. Our view of them was skewed by how we felt about them.

All in all, it's not difficult to conceptualize or explain how addiction might work in terms of brainwashing. This is also an example of how we might achieve it in a relationship—relating it to familiar senses and normalizing it. Using hypnosis and conditioning are the easy bread and butter tools here: Suggest the feelings we want to encourage, and reinforce when we see signs of it. Addiction tends to be self-fulfilling in that it is generally set up as something that feels good and rewarding as well as omnipresent. It feels desirable to seek it out.

In fact, addiction is an issue that tends to come up in brainwashing relationships in general, even inadvertently. Of course we're having intense, pleasurable, erotic experiences, so it stands to reason that we want more and that we have a somewhat unavoidable risk of becoming accustomed to or dependent on our partners. Love is a sort of drug, and we're certainly familiar with what happens especially in the early stages of an intense partnership.

But there is an enormous downside to playing with addiction: Withdrawal. Withdrawal is a very real consequence within any relationship—after all, we get high off of "brain drugs" with our partners all the time—but when we are intentionally using addiction as a tool, this risk skyrockets. Many of us are familiar with the concept of "dom-" or "subdrop" after a scene; the coming down from all the hormones and chemicals being released, which can feel quite unpleasant. When addiction is involved, we are taking advantage of releasing those chemicals in more effective ways and creating a dependency on them. This is very dangerous and we have to be very careful of everyone's mental and emotional states.

Mitigation

It cannot be stressed enough that addiction play is very, very risky, and there is no way to make it safe. The reality is that we do experience intense changes in brain chemistry affects when we engage with people in different ways, and this style of relationship is already primed for addictive behavior—we're doing stuff that feels really good, often with an inherent imbalance of power. Just like with any intense relationship, it can feel like a need; anything that plays with that or attempts to unfold it is going to be quite volatile. There are real consequences to addiction; the normal unpleasantness of missing someone can become intense on a level that is harmful and unacceptable.

Of course, in a consensual brainwashing relationship, we want to minimize the negative effects of any of our play—we definitely don't want to intentionally induce a "drop" or a sense of withdrawal when we aren't around. So we can attempt to mitigate these things in various ways, but it's prudent to remember that we may not be able to completely eliminate it.

Being confident that you will have predictable, consistent contact is very important if addiction is involved in a relationship. This doesn't mean being available 24/7, but certainly setting aside time and being communicative of long gaps. Even the inadvertent expectation of time can be devastating if suddenly dropped. Waiting for a significant amount of time before even introducing addiction play into a relationship is beneficial; finding where a reliable schedule is for communication and getting into good habits and routines together.

Normalizing time apart is also important; you can frame it as healthy and something that helps the upkeep of the relationship. There is a large potential for your partner to feel much "clingier" and needy for your attention, which may not be easy for you to handle. Making sure and monitoring that your partner can function independently when you are not available is essential. You can give them tools to better deal with this sort of thing, as well as drop and withdrawal—such as reminders of you, voice recordings or pictures, or suggestions, tasks, or assignments to keep as psychological tokens.

Identity

Identity is a complicated and nebulous part of psychology. It is what we run into when we attempt to describe ourselves: "Who am I?" It is fluid, shaped by factors such as memories, agency or autonomy, social roles, self-image, beliefs, and experiences. Most people are familiar with the sense that they are a different person than who they were ten years ago, but identity can shift moment-to-moment, as well, depending on our environment and how we are feeling.

Relationships can play a large role in shaping identity—especially in long-term, committed partnerships, we often find that we define ourselves based on the company we choose. We create mutual identities and identities as pairs or groups. Identity, in this case, evolves with another person, with each partner having a role in defining all of the various aspects that make up self-perception. This is doubly true in brainwashing, especially if we are purposefully using self-image as a tool for conditioning.

In fact, tying identity into conditioning and hypnotic suggestion is very powerful. For example, suggesting that someone is easily malleable is attractive and desirable. But suggesting that they are that way because they are who they are (utilizing their personal history and what you know about them—Chapter 6—and "trapping" them with that as well as implying causality—Chapter 8) adds an element of correlation to it in addition to making it something personal and internal.

If you are taking advantage of this on a larger scale, we run into one concept of adding brainwashing as an element of their identity. This is very intense, and may have a tendency to happen naturally over the course of this kind of relationship. It becomes self-reinforcing—when they view and think of themselves, "brainwashed" (and all the aspect that you choose to involve with that) becomes entangled with them. They are a brainwashed person. You shift their definition of their sense of self, which can be quite persistent as well as being an insidious but immense display of control. This can apply to any sort of definition you wish to encourage.

But playing with identity is not just about being additive. It has the potential to be transformative or reductive. In a vanilla relationship, generally both partners influence each other and change together freely. But in brainwashing and edgy play, we may be making changes that define a person, whether that is exerting control over existing aspects, pushing the person to change in different directions, or taking away parts of them, whether temporarily or persistently. Understanding the various aspects of a person's identity is a principal part of being able to play with it; you'll find that there is a lot of variance in what people consider important to their definition of self. You may also consider playing with shifting that sense of importance—what do you want them to focus on as essential aspects of their identity?

Mitigation

While identity changes are common over time and within relationships (and this should be understood as a natural consequence of intimacy), it can be very intense to directly influence them. This is yet another place where neither you nor your partner can trust that they know what they wanted before you started changing them—it's not that they don't genuinely feel the way that they feel, but you both have to make decisions about what is allowable in these cases.

As always, be cautious with what you seek to change. You aren't always going to know what an emotional landmine is in terms of important self-image elements. Neither will your partner. A gentle touch and flexibility goes a long way here. You may consider that starting small is the right thing to do. When playing temporarily, or especially with anything that the subject considers to be a principal aspect of themselves, it may be good to express that it isn't permanent; this serves as both a suggestion as well as assurance that they aren't truly losing something precious to them. Your partner understanding that you have their desires in mind will allow them to let go further and go to more intense places because they trust you.

Sometimes it can be hard to tell what identity changes are a result of brainwashing versus just a result of growing closer. This is unavoidable; hypnosis, conditioning, brainwashing, and everything else are not easily contained magically through suggestion. It must be acknowledged as a risk, but it doesn't mean that you can't work with it. It is better, in many cases, to work with the current state of identity rather than attempt to hearken back to a time or state that doesn't currently exist. Trying to create a "clean slate" will get mixed results; there is no way to truly keep something immutable, including identity and frame of mind. By the same token, people naturally change over time, so trying to use a list of limits or desires that was made a year prior is not going to be accurate, either. There is no such thing as unbiased or unaltered perspective when it comes to relationships. Brainwashing is just one of many things which cause us to evolve—so are intimacy and love. There is no easy answer for "how far is too far" in this scenario. Keep in mind the guidelines from Chapter 2 and be self-analyzing about how healthy the partnership feels

THE BRAINWASHING BOOK

CHAPTER 11: "UNDOING" AND "DEPROGRAMMING"

So what do you do if you want to "deprogram" someone? Maybe you've decided to transition out of brainwashing for some reason, or there are specific behaviors and habits that you've mutually decided aren't serving their purpose anymore. What if you feel something has gone a little too far? How do you "undo" things that have been done?

All of these words are in quotations because thinking in terms of being able to just wipe to a clean slate or reverse a process is not realistic. These are behaviors that have been taught to a person. "Unlearning" isn't a practical or realistic process, even with hypnosis. There are no magic words and no magic state that will do this reliably.

However, all the tools you need to do this have been taught in this book so far. You don't remove conditioned behaviors—you replace them and encourage the natural extinction process, as well as take advantage of a couple more concepts from general psychology.

Why Is It Continuing?

One of the first things to do is to ask yourself why a certain behavior is persisting. One way of looking at this is that a behavior that no longer produces the more positive or familiar response—that is, a behavior which is no longer the "best choice"—will not hold, over time, if there is a better option. On some level, this is a helpful model, but it's oversimplified, so we need to add to it to be more precise. By now, we've discussed at length that one of our best tools for brainwashing (and thus, for un-brainwashing) is being able to understand what is coming into play in terms of environmental reinforcements or punishments, and what associations have been built.

For example, perhaps your partner is conditioned to only orgasm while thinking of you. If we analyze this, of course there is the obvious reinforcement—the expectation of a feeling of pleasure and the pleasure itself. But broken down further, there may be more nuanced associations. That pleasure may take the form of a needed feeling of submission in addition to the physical sensations. Maybe there is an attraction to the nature of it being about orgasm denial. Maybe an emotional attachment to that particular restriction and behavior, because of something intimate and valuable to them about when it was given or memories they have of it being important to them.

Also, not only reinforcements are relevant here—there are also punishments to consider. There is probably a feeling of guilt that comes with the idea of having an orgasm outside of those parameters. Maybe that guilt even comes from experiences they've had where they were scolded for it, or maybe it's more internal. And of course, there could be other elements involved that we won't see at face value.

Sometimes, this will be obvious, and other times, it will require a little bit of discussion and digging. The reality is that we will never be able to know exactly what is going on in someone else's head, and it is key to keep that in mind. The best we can do is be as open and communicative as possible. Often, these conversations can be revealing to both parties—your partner may not realize how much is involved until they start to talk about it. It's essential to be open to how they express themselves, and to listen carefully and respectfully. It's our responsibility to be available to do this in any circumstance we are able when we were involved in the first place, whether it is a natural continuation of a relationship or helping to "clean up" at the end of one.

Extinction

As we've discussed, learned behaviors will tend to naturally become extinct over time if they're not being reinforced. This means that time is your friend, and that in general, most behavioral changes are not so permanent that they will withstand a long period of returning to whatever is considered "normalcy." The key here is that the environment is conducive to this—if the behaviors are continuing to be reinforced, whether inadvertently by yourself, or as a product of circumstance, environment, expectation, or belief, they will tend to be more persistent.

You can do your best to help the process by keeping a careful eye on what your partner is responding to and removing stimuli that are rewarding or punishing them, when possible—potentially, this includes anything set up as an "automatic" reinforcement, such as hypnotic anchors, or behaviors that reward themselves. You can only do so much through hypnosis, and some people in some scenarios will be more receptive than others with just straight suggestions to remove a stimulus.

However, as mentioned earlier, extinction isn't always the most pleasant process. After a period of time of being rewarded for behaving a certain way, it can be uncomfortable and jarring to have that stop. Sometimes, we're able to comfort our partners through this, but other times we have to rely on them to be able to help themselves. The most we can do in this case is to always try to encourage the ability for them to be independent when need be, and to cultivate a sense of self-sufficiency whenever we're able. The best case scenario is when you're able to take advantage of the process of extinction while also replacing various aspects of the behavior or response.

Replacing

If you can't have someone magically unlearn a response, the solution is to change it or replace it with something else. This is done by using the exact same tools we use to train behaviors in the first place; you are, essentially, training another behavior. Sometimes this is called "counterconditioning," but it's no different, functionally, than conditioning itself.

In the previous example of a person conditioned to only orgasm while thinking of you, you have a few options. The first thing you may want to do is work on replacing the guilt that they feel with "disobeying" the conditioning with something more positive. Perhaps giving them a sense of pride in their ability to be well-rounded. Or, maybe a sense of excitement at how many options they have. Have them orgasm while thinking of something else to "prove" to them that it's possible and that it feels good. They may not get rid of the guilt immediately, and that's okay. Learning and conditioning takes time.

As we've discussed, you generally don't want to train behaviors by relying on or using much punishment. So in most cases, it's not the right choice to add in a negative feeling if they perform the initial behavior—there will almost certainly be an urge to at first, and they will probably feel a little guilty or put-down by their impulse anyways. You can assist with that, too, by assuring them that this is a process, not instant. They're not doing anything wrong, they're just following their own natural responses.

We learned through classical conditioning that spontaneous recovery of the original behavior is a possibility—sometimes, it will reemerge, and that's okay. Teaching them not to beat themselves up over it and teaching them about the mechanisms of why behaviors stick, "unstick," and sometimes fluctuate is good to comfort them. They need to understand just as much as you do that none of this is a magical or automatic process.

"What"

Sometimes it takes a bit of thinking about what "behavior" should replace the original. It is good to use the original behavior as a starting point. A lot of the time, being "brainwashed" isn't as easy as pointing to specific behaviors. As we discussed early on, this can be one of the hardest parts of brainwashing—being able to define it in concrete, achievable ways. It is actually a little easier from the perspective of starting with someone who is already conditioned along those lines: You can observe and begin to recognize the patterns of behavior that they or you define that way.

For example, you may want to work on someone's sense of dependency. The first question is: "What are the specific behaviors, external and cognitive, that display a lack of self-sufficiency?" Perhaps they are obsessing over waiting for messages or contact from you or someone else. Perhaps they tend to default to you or someone else making decisions. Perhaps they are starting to define themselves by how another person views them. There are many aspects to what may, on the surface, be a simple idea. Just the same way that you analyze the question, "What makes a brainwashed person?" you have to ask yourself and your partner, "What makes an un-brainwashed person?" It is the same goal-oriented approach.

At this point, it's about finding the underlying behavior or thought patterns and replacing from there. Following this example, perhaps you can give them ways to be distracted from their phone and reward them for that, encourage self-sufficiency and decision making, and cultivate a positive and strong self-image. None of these have to be instantaneous or intense—just a little bit of help towards whatever you consider normalcy.

Don't Do "Therapy"

There is only so much we can do as amateurs. It is often said that erotic and recreational hypnosis and behavior modification is good until we start trying to do "therapy" or "fix" our partners. But where is the line drawn if we're trying to help fix and change detrimental behaviors? Of course, this is all a gray area and there is no easy answer. You and your partner are going to know the most about your own situation, and that includes being able to know when you don't have all the information you need, and when that is a problem.

If there are lasting behavioral changes that are immediately unacceptably distressing and adversely affecting the quality of life, it may be time to seek professional help. Or, if it seems like some patterns are coming from or entangled with a deeper and more troubled place, for example, other areas of life or their personal history. We can do our best to support our partners and help them in whatever ways we have available to us. When in doubt, err on the side of caution, and especially if it seems that the tools we are using are not effective in the long run.

IN CONCLUSION

Even with everything I've written here, the broad and the specific, we only scratch the surface on a lot of these concepts. However, I hope I've been able to shed some light on a wide breadth of ideas and inspire you to take them, dive further if you so desire, and apply them in your fun and kinky play.

I have found that at a certain point in trying to further my hypnosis skills, I had to branch out to really learn more. For me, this means exploring adjacent topics in psychology, sociology, linguistics, even spirituality and elsewhere. I strongly urge you to do the same—you may find that your existing knowledge creates a helpful frame of reference with which to synergize to create something greater. I hope that this book helps you find ideas to research—it all can be applied to kink, sometimes in ways that we don't initially expect. Knowledge, in this case, quite literally is power.

Brainwashing is an enormously fulfilling kink that also happens to be quite broad. It creates bonds between people that feel deep and real, and it is something that evolves with relationships. It can mold to and take the shape of the desires of the participants. For you, this might be about using the model that I have put forth as-is, or it might be using it as a springboard to find new depths and methods. Feel free to do what feels natural and right to you and your partners—as long as you approach it ethically and with a desire for mutual enjoyment.

Most of all, thank you for supporting me through this long process and by picking up a copy for yourself. It means the world to me that I can create something worthwhile, especially for the community that I dreamed endlessly about existing when I was young. But even in my wildest fantasies, I never thought I would be doing something like this. Thank you to everyone who had an influence on me along the way.

Now go and have fun!

GLOSSARY

BDSM: An acronym for "Bondage and Discipline, Dominance and Submission, and Sadism and Masochism." Often interchangeable with "kink."

Bottom: The "receiving" partner in a certain kinky activity, and not necessarily dominant or submissive.

Brainwashing: A kinky activity that allows us to set and achieve goals with our partner through the use of various methods and principles including operant conditioning, classical conditioning, hypnosis, and more.

Classical conditioning: Initially "discovered" by Ivan Pavlov, it is a form of learning that involves pairing stimuli and responses.

Dominant: The partner who has power or control over the other, whether in roleplay or reality.

D/s: An abbreviation for "dominance and submission." Often describes a style of relationship.

Hypnosis: A broad term that encompasses a set of practices that may or may not involve suggestion, altered states, and/or focus. It also refers to the "trance" state within these practices.

Hypnotist: The partner who is guiding, controlling, or otherwise leading a hypnotic interaction. Not necessarily dominant or submissive.

Kink: Erotic activity outside of "traditional" sexuality, often encompassing fetishism, sex, or nonsexual intimacy.

Negotiation: The process and conversations in which all parties involved are ensured to be consenting to kinky activities and understand the depth of what is on the table.

NLP: Short for "Neurolinguistic Programming"; refers to a model and set of practices initially put forth by Richard Bandler and John Grinder. It attempts to study effective therapists and explain what they do that is so useful to create persistent change.

Operant conditioning: A principle studied by B.F. Skinner and many others, it is the way an organism learns behaviors through the use of intentional or unintentional reinforcement or punishment.

Play: Catch-all term for kinky activity of all sorts, whether sexual or nonsexual.

RACK: An acronym for "Risk-Aware Consensual Kink," which attempts to describe a model for having safer kink interactions through risk awareness, acceptance, and mitigation.

Scene: A self-contained kink encounter with a beginning, middle, and end. Scenes are a way for partners to express eroticism and may be pre-planned or spontaneous.

Subject: The partner who is being guided, controlled, or otherwise led in a hypnotic interaction. Not necessarily dominant or submissive.

Submissive: The partner who gives up power or control to the other, whether in roleplay or reality. In some models, the submissive is seen as the one who holds power in the relationship by nature of giving their consent and submission.

Switch: A person who enjoys both the "Top" and "bottom" roles, and/or the "Dominant" and "submissive" roles.

Top: The "giving" partner in a certain kinky activity, and not necessarily dominant or submissive.

THE BRAINWASHING BOOK

BIBLIOGRAPHY

Aoki, K. (1999). Introduction: Language Is a Virus. Retrieved from https://repository.law.miami.edu/umlr/vol53/iss4/21/.

Bandler, R. (2008). *Guide to Trance-formation: How to Harness the Power of Hypnosis to Ignite Effortless and Lasting Change*. Deerfield Beach, FL: Health Communications, Inc.

Bandler, R., & Grinder, J. (1975). *The Structure of Magic I: A Book About Language and Therapy*. Palo Alto, CA: Science and Behavior Books.

Britannica, T. E. of E. (n.d.). Associative learning. Retrieved from http://www.britannica.com/topic/associative-learning.

Cherry, K. (2019, September 24). The Psychology of How People Learn. Retrieved from http://www.verywellmind.com/what-is-learning-2795332.

Coates, G. (n.d.). Watzlawick's Five Axioms. Retrieved from http://www.wanterfall.com/Communication-Watzlawick's-Axioms.htm.

Forms of Pavlovian Conditioning. (n.d.). Retrieved from http://www.indiana.edu/~p1013447/dictionary/pavfrm.htm.

Hochman, G., & Erev, I. (2013, December). The partial-reinforcement extinction effect and the contingent-sampling hypothesis. Retrieved from https://www.ncbi.nlm.nih.gov/pubmed/23595350.

Kohn, A. (2018). *Punished by Rewards: the Trouble with Gold Stars, Incentive Plans, as, Praise, and Other Bribes.* Houghton Mifflin Harcourt Trade & Reference Publishers.

Lankton, S. R., & Lankton, C. H. (2014). *The Answer Within: A Clinical Framework of Ericksonian Hypnotherapy.* Routledge.

Pryor, K. (2000). The Ten Laws of Shaping. Retrieved from http://www.clickertraining.com/node/299.

Pryor, K. (2018). *Don't Shoot the Dog!: The New Art of Teaching and Training.* Dorking, Surrey: Ringpress Books Ltd.

Roffman, A. E. (2008). Men are Grass: Bateson, Erickson, Utilization and Metaphor. *American Journal of Clinical Hypnosis*, 50(3). doi: 10.1080/00029157.2008.10401627

Schachtman, T. R., Walker, J. R., & Fowler, S. R. (2011). Effects of Conditioning in Advertising. *Associative Learning and Conditioning Theory.* doi: 10.1093/acprof:oso/9780199735969.003.0157

Shrestha, P. (2019, June 16). Operant Conditioning Definition and Concepts. Retrieved from http://www.psychestudy.com/behavioral/learning-memory/operant-conditioning/definition-concepts.

Sijll, J. V. (n.d.). Cinematic Storytelling: Dynamic Metaphors. Retrieved from http://www.writersstore.com/cinematic-storytelling-dynamic-metaphors/.

Skinner, B. F. (2014). Science and Human Behavior. Retrieved from www.bfskinner.org/newtestsite/wp-content/uploads/2014/02/ScienceHumanBehavior.pdf.

ABOUT THE AUTHOR

sleepingirl is a queer writer, presenter, and podcaster with a decade of real-life erotic hypnosis experience on both sides of the "pocket watch." She has a lifelong passion for the cerebral and intimate and has taught at kink events across the United States. Find her on Twitter @h_sleepingirl, Tumblr @h-sleepingirl, FetLife @sleepingirl. She hosts a podcast on hypnokink with her brainwashed partner: "Two Hyp Chicks."

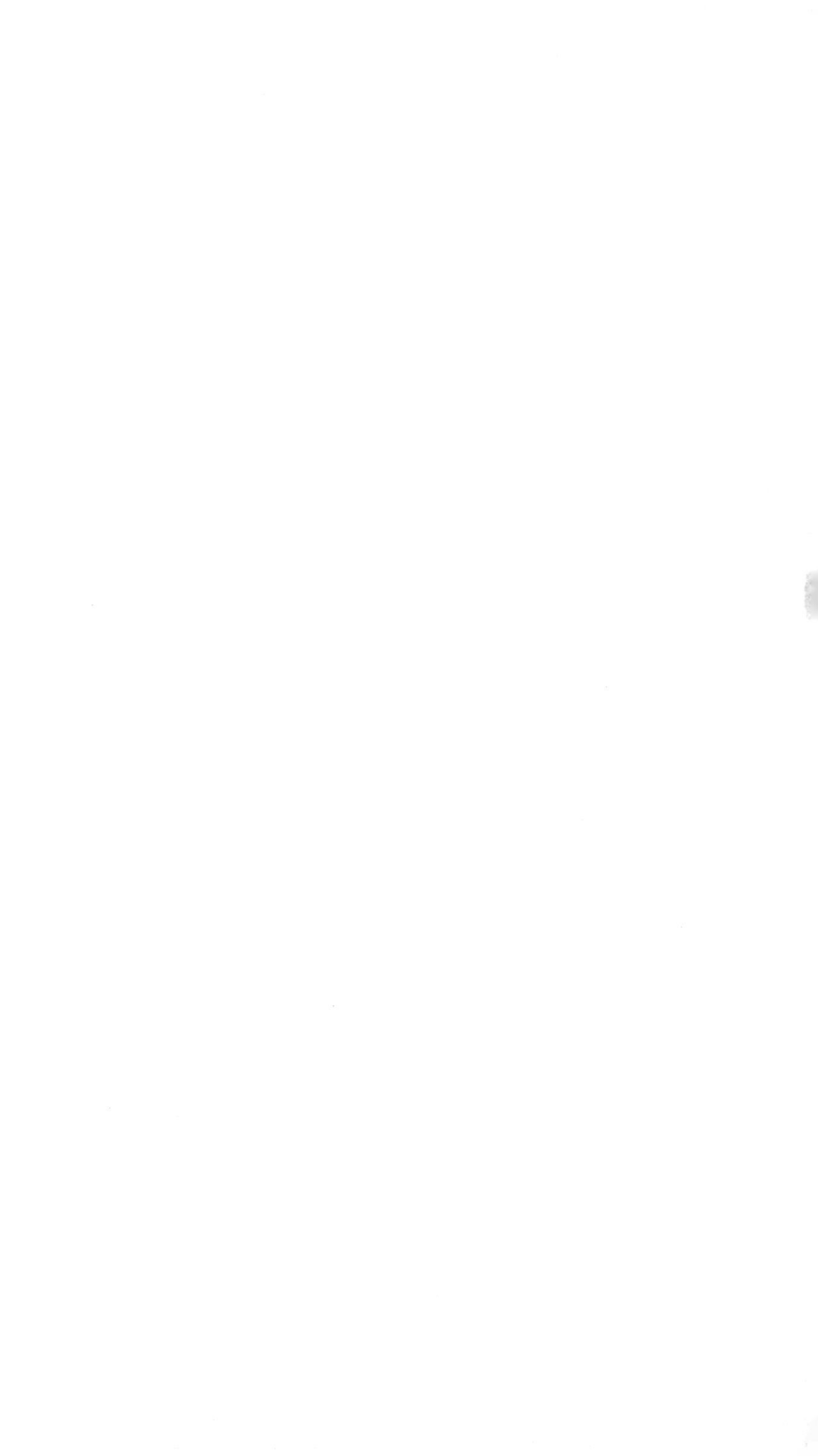

Printed in Great Britain
by Amazon